Dr. Karen Drake's

Book of Hope

A Theopathic Guide to Healing

Karen E. Drake, D. Min., T.M.D.

Phoenix University of Theology International

Dr. Karen Drake's

Book of Hope

Copyright 2015 by Dr. Karen E. Drake

Published by

Phoenix University of Theology International
Box 86054
Phoenix, AZ 85080
email: PhoenixUTI@gmail.com

Cover design: Carrie Wachsmann, Win Wachsmann

All rights reserved. No portion of this book may be reproduced in any form without the written permission of the publisher.

Printed in USA

TABLE OF CONTENTS

Accolades 5
Acknowledgment 7
Dedication 9
Introduction 13
Sanoviv Miracles 19
History and Testimony ~ A Day I Will Never Forget 41
Healing Prayers 57
Treatment and Decisions 61
Skepticism 71
What I Did and Why I Did It 75
Daily Regimen 77
Homeopathic Remedies 83
Botanical Herbs 85
Drainage 87
Foods and Their Health Benefits 91
Understand Your Body -
With Spiritual and Twenty-first Century References 97

Mental Attitude 105
Diet 113
When is Abstinence Required 119
Wine and Spirits 125
The Dangers of Food Additives 129
Water 137
Exercise 145
Sunlight 151
Rest 157
Meditation 163
Our Body's pH Level and How It Affects Our Health 167
Alkaline-Forming Foods 171
Dental Focus 177
Coffee Enema Cleanse 183
Benefits of Coffee Enema Cleanse 185
References 187

ACCOLADES

Deepest gratitude to my loving family…

My parents, Robert and Eileen Cook, raised me in a Christian home, and saw to it that I was educated at St. John's Lutheran School in Arnold, Missouri. There, I learned to trust in God—Father, Son, and Holy Spirit—Who became my constant Companion and best Friend. My faith in God and appreciation for His blessings instilled in me as a child sustained me through this life-threatening illness.

My father loves the outdoors. He taught me to fish from the creek bank, hunt the woods for wild mushrooms and the pastures for blackberries. He taught me to appreciate being alone in the silent beauty of nature and respect all that God provided for our nourishment and enjoyment.

My mother always tried a natural approach before racing off to the physician for every little ailment. She used a hot rag for an earache and ice for a burn—teaching me the simple truth that natural cures can be administered safely and effectively at home.

My paternal grandparents, Walter Emory and Nora Cook, depended on the bounty of the land to sustain them. I will always remember the trips to the meadow where grandma selected wild plants for our dinner...the hours she spent picking out wild hickory nuts for her wonderful baked goods. Also, the time spent with grandpa, fishing from the creek bank, tending to his animals, and listening to his stories of times past while he barbecued over an open fire. These experiences left an indelible impression on me—imparting an appreciation for God's natural provision.

My maternal grandparents, Theodore and Ruth Noll, on whose farm I had the good fortune to be raised. Their long days spent working in the fields raising crops for a living taught me the value of hard work, the importance of family, and enveloped me with an unalterable sense of security. I will never forget the fragrance of the freshly-tilled earth, the delight in eating vegetables right in the field, or the smells of the harvest. Never was a meal eaten without thanking God for His bounty and provision. Nor would a day go by without experiencing the beauty of God's creation.

ACKNOWLEDGEMENT

There are many people who have encouraged the writing of this book; however, there are several to whom I must give special recognition and thanks.

Firstly, my husband, Richard, who more than anyone else saw the vision of *"hope"* my experience could offer others afflicted with this life-threatening illness. He, therefore, diligently pursued me to record what I learned during this experience and instructed me in the wisdom (strength) and comfort offered throughout the Word of God.

Secondly, Barbara Watts, of *Quick Study, Good Friends, Inc.,* is indeed a gift from God. She offered to edit this work and committed countless hours of her precious time critiquing it. It is through her devotion and creative genius that my experience has been transformed into a publishable work.

Finally, my beloved friends and neighbors—Mrs. Ethel Meals, Demetra Foster, Maurice Craig, and Jeanne Muriah—for their time devoted to proofreading and the priceless hours spent encouraging me throughout this ordeal.

DEDICATION

First and foremost I dedicate this book to my Heavenly Father, without whom I could not have survived my battle with breast cancer. He gave me the willpower and perseverance to continue searching for a natural ap- proach to beat cancer and restore my body to health. His word assured me that He would give me wisdom in my search. James 1:5 says: *"If any of you lack wisdom, let him ask of God, who giveth to all men liberally and upbraideth not, and it shall be given him."* Then Ezekiel 4:7 speaks of God's intention for the trees and plants He created *"the fruit thereof shall be for food and the leaf thereof for medicine."*

My experience taught me, what the Apostle Paul meant in his letter to the Philippians, Philippians 4:13 *"I can do all things through Christ which strengtheneth me"*. Without the strength that I received through my faith in Christ,

I fear I would have been overwhelmed by the magnitude of doubt and skepticism constantly challenging me to take the contemporary medical ap- proach rather than to seek the natural way to health. By His grace and mercy I was healed.

Secondly - to my precious husband, Richard, who respected and defended my decision to treat cancer with a holistic approach. He encouraged me to stand on what I believed and prayerfully stood with me day after day throughout the long and frustrating two years as we battling not only the cancer, but also; those that thought I was insane to disobey the medical doctors. It was through his insistence that I journal my experiences and the miraculous ways in which God moved to restore my health that this book has been written.

Finally - my deepest gratitude to all those that prayed for me to recover. It was their faith and encour- agement that gave me hope. As the Bible instructs in James 5:14 ***"Is any sick among you? let him call for the elders of the church; and let them pray over him, anointing him with oil in the name of the Lord".*** I never would have known how many friends I had and how deeply their love went, if I had not been challenged with cancer. They offered not only physical strength but also financial support when necessary. If I hadn't put my life and recovery in God's hands, I would have missed out on all the miracles.

God laid it on the hearts of dear friends, John and Sharon, Jim and Nellie and Bobby and Virginia Parker to help financially when I had no other means. God miraculously made me aware of Sanoviv, the medical facility in Mexico, where I received treatment, and laid it on our friends John and Sharon's hearts to fund my treatment there.

God put the right people into my life just when I needed them, Joyce Rathburn, at Sanoviv, who encouraged me to read, Psalms 27 which assured me that even if everyone else would forsake me, "Then the LORD will take care of me" and to "Wait on the LORD; Be of good courage, And He shall strengthen your heart; Wait, I say, on the LORD!".

Last but certainly not least, God arranged for me to receiving treatment at Sanoviv when Jon and Esther were there. He also laid it on their hearts to volunteer to pay for my surgery and the additional expenses of the vitamins and supplements that I would need during my recovery.

I will never forget the humbling feeling of having so many, care so deeply for me. Such love I could have never imagined. Thank you all!

GALATIANS 3:26

For ye are all the children of God by faith in Christ Jesus.

INTRODUCTION

Even as a child, I always wanted to help others. I felt compelled to make everyone I encountered smile—to bring some joy or gladness to their day. For a long time, I actually believed my Mother and Father named me Karen because I was to be a caring (Kar'en) person.

I dreamed of becoming a missionary then thought of being a teacher. Circumstances, however, prevented my educational dreams from materializing until my life's experiences, the highs and lows, prepared me to follow my dreams.

For many years, I satisfied my desire to help others and make a difference in the world by working in the medical field while tithing my income to help those less fortunate. God's Word is very specific about tithing. Deuteronomy 2:16: *"You shall bring your...tithes and the offering of your hands, and your vows and your freewill offerings, and the firstlings of your herd and of your flock."* Malachi 3:7-9 (Amplified Bible) also warns what to expect if we do not tithe: *"Return to me, and I will return to you, says the Lord of hosts. But you say, How shall we return? Will a man rob or defraud God? …. But you say, In what way do we rob or defraud You? [You have withheld your] tithes and offerings. You are cursed with the curse, for you are robbing Me, even this whole nation."*

I know we are to use our lives and our income for more than our own existence and pleasure. Colossians 3:12-17 describes how we ought to live our lives: *"Therefore, as the elect of God, holy and beloved, put on tender mercies, kindness, humility, meekness, longsuffering; bearing with one another, and forgiving one another, if anyone has a complaint against another; even as Christ forgave you, so you also must do. But above all these things put on love (charity), which is the bond of perfection. And let the peace of God rule in your hearts, to which also you were called in one body; and be thankful. Let the word of Christ dwell in you richly in all wisdom, teaching and admonishing one another in psalms and hymns and spiritual songs, singing with grace in your hearts to the Lord. And whatever you do in word or deed, do all in the name of the Lord Jesus, giving thanks to God the Father through Him."*

There was always a gnawing in my spirit that my work as a medical assistant was just not doing enough. I tried to encourage others and share the Word of God—praying with the patients and putting inspirational Scriptures on every patient's receipts each day. Then, one day, I came across a message in my daily inspirational calendar that touched my spirit. I began to pray it every day: "Lord, help me to fulfill my potential." The Word of God tells us in Matthew 7:7 *"Ask and it shall be given you; seek, and ye shall find; knock and it shall be opened unto you."* I believed God would direct my path; His Word promised He would.

One Monday morning in late August 1998, I was awakened, hearing a voice saying: "Be a doctor." I felt God was answering my prayer by directing my path. I had never been to college or taken the college entrance examination. Now, in middle-age, it seemed an unlikely possibility. However, I felt so strongly about what I had heard that I went that very morning and signed up for classes at a nearby college—Union University in Jackson, Tennessee. God is great! Not only was I accepted into the pre-med program but the classes actually started that night! My counselor scheduled my college placement tests for the following Saturday. Amazingly, after being away from school for so many years, I passed the tests! It was awesome how God opened the doors when I followed His instructions.

In order to complete my Bachelor's program as quickly as possible, I moved to St. Louis, Missouri, and stayed with my Aunt Alice—taking accelerated courses at Logan Chiropractic College. I had heard of a new program being offered in Phoenix, Arizona, at the College of Integrative Medicine—combined courses in medical and naturopathic studies. I wanted to be one of the first to enroll. I was on a mission and had no time to waste!

After the first semester at the College of Integrative Medicine, I realized that my desire [and I believe my calling] was to focus more on health and healing through natural means than on the standard medical and pharmacological approach. Therefore, I transferred to Southwest Naturopathic College in Tempe, Arizona, to continue my studies.

While attending school in Arizona, I married an amazing man. He is a minister, teacher, and theologian. I have never met anyone like him! He is awesome! His unwavering faith in God and total commitment to serving the Lord, coupled with his deep understanding of the Word of God and compassion for his fellowman, inspired me so much that I actually prayed to be like him. My marriage caused me to reevaluate my educational goals. Once again, I changed my focus—this time to Theology, majoring in the healing principals directed by Scripture. 2 Timothy 2:15: *"Study to shew thyself approved unto God, a workman that needeth not to be ashamed, rightly dividing the word of truth."* Now I knew I was on the right track and on the way to fulfilling my potential!

In 2003, I received my Master's Degree in Ministry from Phoenix Theological Seminary then went on to attain my Doctorate in Theopathic Health and Healing in 2008 from Phoenix University of Theology.

This unique course of study teaches Christian, spiritual, biblical, and natural perspectives on health and healing. The focus is on the natural healing process – walking in God's healing power, embracing a life of divine health, and having a greater impact and influence on one's own "path" to health and healing "God's Way."

CHAPTER 1

SANOVIV MIRACLES

During most of 2006, my battle with breast cancer consisted of natural approaches to treatment in the belief my body was designed by God to heal itself if given the proper nutrition, diet, and exercise along with the proper mental attitude. The Word of God tells us to pray and have faith in the healing grace of our Lord and Savior Jesus Christ, because it is through His grace, not our works, that we are saved. Ephesians 2:8 tells us: *"For by grace are ye saved through faith; and that not of yourselves: it is the gift of God,"* and 2 Timothy 1:9: *"Who hath saved us, and called us with an holy calling, not according to our works, but according to his own purpose and grace, which was given us in Christ Jesus before the world began…"*

I discovered the lump in January and did everything I

could afford to restore my body to health. By November, however, the tumor was still detectable.

My husband and I were out of money, unable to continue purchasing the expensive vitamins and supplements that had been so much a part of my treatment. We decided, even though our resources were limited, I should take one final trip to Melbourne, Florida, to see Dr. Jonathan Clark, and get a reading on how the cancer was responding thus far. The report was encouraging! My body was obviously reacting favorably to everything I was doing—the tumor had shrunken from the size of my thumb to the size of the tip of my little finger! But still...it was there, and there was no more money to purchase products.

I had *confessed* it—now I had to *believe* (even though things looked a little bleak right then) that my recovery was completely *in God's hands*. Hebrews 13:5 tells us: "*... Be content with such things as ye have: for he hath said, I will never leave thee, nor forsake thee.*"

It wasn't until all our financial resources were exhausted that I stopped trying to find the cure and put my total faith in God. There is no doubt that everything I did was beneficial to my recovery; but in the end, *it was all God*! It was time I trusted totally in Him and not my research or financial resources.

I prayerfully spent every available moment in Florida walking on the warm sandy beaches, soaking up the balmy sun's rays, and enjoying the wonderful ocean breeze for the last time. I knew this was the final stage of treatment as I had known it. My husband was in Tennessee praying for God's guidance while I was in Florida praying the same; both of us knowing that God would show us the way. Matthew 18:19 assures us: *"Again I say unto you, That if two of you shall agree on earth as touching any thing that they shall ask, it shall be done for them of my Father which is in heaven."*

What an awesome God we serve! By the time I returned home, our prayers had been answered. While I was in Florida, a close friend called and told my husband, Richard, an incredible story of a man and his wife that he had encountered by chance on three different occasions while lecturing in Ohio. He said after the third encounter, he felt God was trying to show him something and he thought of me. The woman had terminal cancer, was put on morphine, and sent home to die. Unwilling to accept this death sentence, her husband equipped a private plane and flew her to a hospital in Mexico—where he had learned they use alternative medical treatment for cancer patients and claim remarkable results. Their story was that she went home from that treatment after two weeks free of cancer!

Our friend called to give us the couple's phone number so we could talk to them. As he was giving Richard the number, he saw the couple approaching him in the hotel. He offered the phone to them so they could speak directly to my husband. The story was very encouraging except for one thing—the treatment was expensive, and we were out of money.

After arriving home in Dallas, our friend John shared his story with his lovely wife, Sharon—they "felt led" to help us financially. John informed Richard they were sending a check to cover the trip and two weeks' of treatment. Remember the promise of God in Luke 6:38: ***I shall cause men to give into your bosom.***

God had made a way when there seemed to be no way—just like the song says:

God Will Make A Way
        Words and Music by Don Moen

God will make a way,
    Where there seems to be no way
        He works in ways we cannot see

He will make a way for me
He will be my guide
Hold me closely to His side
With love and strength for each new day
He will make a way, He will make a way.
By a roadway in the wilderness, He'll lead me
And rivers in the desert will I see
Heaven and earth will fade
But His Word will still remain
He will do something new today.

<u>Proverbs 3:6</u>

"In all thy ways acknowledge him, and he shall direct thy paths."

God put this man with his amazing testimony into John's life at just the right moment then laid it on John's heart to pay the $1,000 per day for my treatment. It is magnificent how God so profoundly answered our prayer, in His timing.

I knew in my heart and soul this was going to be the treatment that cured me. I thanked God with every ounce of my energy and told everyone I met about God's answer to our prayers. I was on *Cloud Nine*, confident that this was God-ordained. 1 Chronicles 16:8 instructs us to: ***"Give thanks unto the LORD, call upon his name, make known his deeds among the people."***

Several days before I was to leave for Mexico, I had a dream about being at the hospital which was like a dingy, barren fortress—all enclosed and frightening. Apparently, I was a bit more apprehensive about the trip than I realized, for my mind to have conjured up such a thought. I was inspired by remembering the Scripture from Joshua 1:7-9 ***"...Be thou strong and very courageous,...that thou mayest prosper withersoever thou goest. This book...thou shalt meditate therein day and night, that thou mayest observe to do according to all that is written therein: for then thou shalt make thy way prosperous, and then thou shalt have good success. Have not I commanded thee? Be strong and of a good courage; be not afraid, neither be thou dismayed: for the LORD thy God is with thee whithersoever thou goest."***

The very next night, I had another dream. Again, I was at the hospital. However, this time, it was like a beautiful mansion—pristine and bright. I was in front of this marvelous estate saying farewell to an elegant lady; it appeared we had been close friends. As we hugged goodbye, she said that she wanted to adopt me, but I would need to change my name to Rosemary Rothschild. I remember waking up at that moment saying out loud: "Rosemary Rothschild" and feeling empowered by such an elegant name. The Bible tells us that God speaks to us in dreams and visions. In Psalm 50:7-15, He assures us He is our God and everything is His: *"Hear, O my people, and I will speak; ... I am God, even thy God... For every beast of the forest is mine, and the cattle upon a thousand hills. ... for the world is mine, and the fullness thereof...call upon me in the day of trouble: I will deliver thee, and thou shalt glorify me."*

What peace to know that God, our Heavenly Father, has limitless resources; and, therefore, we as His heirs have the same. Romans 8:15 says *"...You have not received a spirit that makes you fearful slaves. Instead, you received God's Spirit when he adopted you as his own children. Now we call him, Abba, Father."*

In Isaiah 62:2, we read that we will receive a new name: *"And thou shalt be called by a new name, which the mouth of the LORD shall name."*

Galatians 4:4-7 speaks directly about our inheritance: *"... God sent forth his Son, ...To redeem them that were under the law, that we might receive the adoption of sons. And because ye are sons, God hath sent forth the Spirit of his Son into your hearts, crying, Abba, Father. Wherefore thou art no more a servant, but a son; and if a son, then an heir of God through Christ."*

As children of God, we need not worry, we need only believe as it says in Mark 9:23 *"Jesus said unto him, If thou canst believe, all things are possible to him that believeth."*

Our friend, John, was financing the hospital expenses, and God continued to provide for the rest of our needs by encouraging others to give of their resources. Luke 6:38 tells us *"Give, and it shall be given unto you; good measure, pressed down, and shaken together, and running over, shall men give into your bosom. For with the same measure that ye mete withal it shall be measured to you again."*

The airfare for the trip to Mexico was made possible by my parents with a $1,500 Christmas gift, and our church took up a collection of $1,400 which supplied all the rest of what was needed to get to the hospital in Mexico. I believed whatever happened on this trip was the will of God—He was ordering the circumstances. In Matthew 6:25-34, basically, we are told to take it one day at a time and leave the cares of the world up to God:

"Therefore I say unto you, Take no thought for your

life, what ye shall eat, or what ye shall drink; nor yet for your body, what ye shall put on. Is not the life more than meat, and the body than raiment? Behold the fowls of the air: for they sow not, neither do they reap, nor gather into barns; yet your heavenly Father feedeth them. Are ye not much better than they? Which of you by taking thought can add one cubit unto his stature? And why take ye thought for raiment? Consider the lilies of the field, how they grow; they toil not, neither do they spin: And yet I say unto you, That even Solomon in all his glory was not arrayed like one of these. Wherefore, if God so clothe the grass of the field, which today is, and tomorrow is cast into the oven, shall he not much more clothe you, O ye of little faith? Therefore take no thought, saying, What shall we eat? or, What shall we drink? or, Wherewithal shall we be clothed? For your heavenly Father knoweth that ye have need of all these things. But seek ye first the kingdom of God, and his righteousness; and all these things shall be added unto you. Take therefore no thought for the morrow: for the morrow shall take thought for the things of itself. Sufficient unto the day is the evil thereof."

My flight landed in San Diego, California, on Tuesday, January 23, 2007—two days short of one year from the day I first found the lump in my breast. I had come a long way since the oncologist, in essence, pronounced my six-month death sentence. From there, the *Sanoviv* shuttle drove me the thirty-mile trip to Santa Rosa just south of Tijuana. Traveling was easy. The hospital instructed me to bring nothing to the hospital: no clothes; no shoes; no cosmetics; no toiletries—they provide everything. It was as Matthew 6:25-34 says: **"*Take no thought for your life, what ye shall eat, or what ye shall drink; nor yet for your body, what ye shall put on.*"**

Since I had not done a great deal of traveling outside the United States, the trip through Customs and into Mexico was a bit intimidating. People were not friendly; and since I don't speak Spanish, I felt vulnerable. As we pulled into the garrison-looking, walled hospital and stopped at the huge iron gates awaiting the guard to allow us access; I had a flashback to my first dream and imagined the prison-type environment that might be awaiting me inside those walls.

Praise the Lord, the second dream was accurate! As the shuttle passed through the gates, which quickly closed behind us, I observed this beautiful stucco facility with more windows than walls, encompassed in an elegant garden setting complete with waterfalls, stone walkways, statuary, and magnificent flowers and greenery.

I had heard about extravagant, luxury hospitals where the rich and famous go for rest and healing. Well, this was one of those places! The main building was originally Levi Strauss' sprawling, marble mansion, situated on the rocky cliffs overlooking the Pacific. It has now been transformed into a luxury hospital with the same sense of affluence and attention to details.

The initial tour and registration process was thorough but lacking any real sense of warmth. Everyone seemed very professional and all business. However, since I had been raised in a large affectionate family and live in a small town in Tennessee where I know all my neighbors, this place seemed rather cold. I felt like I needed a hug.

After registration, I was shown to my suite which was gorgeous—well, at least the view was gorgeous. The balcony overlooked the Pacific, and the splendidly landscaped pool and spa areas were just below my window. I loved it! The bedroom drawers were filled with everything I was to wear, and the bathroom was fully stocked with all the necessary toiletries. I understood the concept that in this controlled environment everyone wore the same thing, so as to avoid any sensitivity or reactions to fabric, detergent, or perfumes. But, somehow, it seemed a little bit like a *Twilight Zone* movie, with everyone dressed identically.

I changed into tan cotton sweats and therapeutic sandals and went to the main floor to start my treatments. There is a pleasant waiting area in the main lobby where everyone congregates as they wait to be escorted by the physicians and therapists to whatever treatment they will be receiving. They don't let you wait long, so there isn't much time to get to know the other patients.

My first day was pretty awkward. It actually took about twenty-four hours before I understood the routine and found out where everything was located. I decided to make it my personal quest to prevent anyone else from having such an uncomfortable first day, so I greeted every new patient and familiarized them with the things that had baffled me initially. It wasn't that difficult to meet everyone, since I have never met a stranger and the hospital only accommodates forty patients at any one time.

That Wednesday evening, the hospital had given permission for the patients to hold a prayer meeting in the library. The atmosphere throughout the entire hospital changed—everyone was excited about getting together. It was as if God had planned for this many Christians to be together at the hospital at the same time, praising and worshiping Him, giving strength and encouragement to each other. Jon and Esther lead the meeting with a Scripture reading and prayer, then we all sang hymns and prayed for one another. Everyone told their particular story, and we all became instant family. Matthew 12:50 tells us *"For whosoever shall do the will of my Father which is in heaven, the same is my brother, and sister, and mother."* From that point on, even the physicians and therapists prayed and discussed Scripture during treatments.

The hospital is great. Every patient has a schedule for their daily activities, and the appointments flow like a finely-tuned machine. There is little, if any, waiting time. Each day began at six a.m. with a warm cup of lemon water and cayenne pepper; one half hour later, four ounces of wheat grass; then off to exercise class and meditation before breakfast which consists of oats, nuts, and fruit. The morning hours are spent with testing and lab work, then lunch. Afternoons are spent in therapy, some more enjoyable than others, like massage, facial, manicure, sauna, and pool time. Dinner is promptly at six p.m. The meals are all served buffet-style with all the salad, sprouts, and seeds one can eat and, of course, hands full of vitamins. Evenings are reserved for lecture and instruction classes. Finally, one more therapy—then off to bed by 10:15 p.m.

Over the course of several days, I had extensive diagnostic testing, lab work, x-rays and more therapies than

I could count. On Friday, the test results were in and the physicians were ready with their medical evaluations. I expected them to tell me that the diet, supplements, and treatment they were providing would cure the cancer. So, I was disheartened when they recommended surgical removal of the cancerous tumor. I knew God had arranged the circumstances that had gotten me to **Sanoviv**, and I believed He would continue to provide whatever was necessary for my healing.

I told the physician my story of how a friend sponsored my treatment and that I had no money for surgery. He explained why the tumor needed to be removed, told me the exact cost of the surgery ($13,950), and said he would continue with the treatment schedule as originally outlined and pray for the best.

That evening, I called my husband and told him of the physician's recommendation for surgery. My husband is awesome—his faith never wavers. He assured me that he was confident God would make a way if surgery was indeed what I needed. Together, we prayed for God's will to be done and that He strengthen my faith, recalling Hebrews 11:1 and 6 *"Now faith is the substance of things hoped for, the evidence of things not seen. But without faith it is impossible to please him: for he that cometh to God must believe that he is, and that he is a rewarder of them that diligently seek him."*

After speaking with my husband, I also called my parents to let them know how the treatment was going and to tell them the physician recommended surgery at a cost of $13,950. My parents were skeptical of any treatment that was not standard medical treatment and performed in the United States. So, when my Mother told me that I should come home and have the surgery where my insurance would pay for it, I was not surprised. It just confirmed that it was God Who would be ordering the circumstances for my recovery.

The next morning the patients had scheduled a worship service. I was asked to be prepared to read a Scripture. Not sure which Scripture to read, I asked one of the patients that had completed their treatment and was leaving the hospital before the service to suggest one. She said her favorite Scripture was Psalm 27:

"The LORD is my light and my salvation; whom shall I fear? The LORD is the strength of my life; of whom shall I be afraid? When the wicked, even mine enemies and my foes, came upon me to eat up my flesh, they stumbled and fell. Though an host should encamp against me, my heart shall not fear: though war should rise against me, in this will I be confident. One thing have I

desired of the LORD, that will I seek after; that I may dwell in the house of the LORD all the days of my life, to behold the beauty of the LORD, and to enquire in his temple. For in the time of trouble he shall hide me in his pavilion: in the secret of his tabernacle shall he hide me; he shall set me up upon a rock. And now shall mine head be lifted up above mine enemies round about me: therefore will I offer in his tabernacle sacrifices of joy; I will sing, yea, I will sing praises unto the LORD. Hear, O LORD, when I cry with my voice: have mercy also upon me, and answer me. When thou saidst, Seek ye my face; my heart said unto thee, Thy face, LORD, will I seek. Hide not thy face far from me; put not thy servant away in anger: thou hast been my help; leave me not, neither forsake me, O God of my salvation. When my father and my mother forsake me, then the LORD will take me up. Teach me thy way, O LORD, and lead me in a plain path, because of mine enemies. Deliver me not over unto the will of mine enemies: for false witnesses are risen up against me, and such as breathe out cruelty. I had fainted, unless I had believed to see the goodness of the LORD in the land of the living. Wait on the LORD: be of good courage, and he shall strengthen thine heart: wait, I say, on the LORD."

That Scripture spoke to me in a way that I had never

before known. This day, when I am searching for provision for a surgery that I need, the Lord instructs me in the final verse: *Wait on the LORD: be of good courage, and he shall strengthen thine heart: wait, I say, on the LORD."*

Instruction to be patient—something I have never been very good at. I read the entire chapter of Psalm 27 during the service Sunday morning. I don't know if it affected anyone else the way it did me; but I will never forget how God used another friend to lead me to just the right Scripture at just the right moment in my life.

On Monday morning, January 29, I was passing one of the treatment lounges when I saw Esther sitting all alone taking her daily IV (intravenous) treatment. Esther and her husband were the patients that put together the Wednesday evening prayer meeting and the Sunday service. Esther's husband, Jon, plays the guitar which made singing hymns much more enjoyable. As I approached Esther to say hello, she asked: *"When will you be having your surgery?"* I responded that I would not be having surgery. She asked: *"Why not?"* I explained that I did not have the money for surgery. She asked: *"How much is it?"* I told her: $13,950. She threw her hands up into the air, IV tubes dangling from her arm, and exclaimed: *"Well, do it girl. I will pay for it. I have my checkbook with me."* I must have just stood there dumbfounded by what she was volunteering to do, because the next thing I heard was her saying: *"Well! Go! Go! Set it up with the doctor."* With tears in my eyes and feeling more blessed than I have ever felt in my entire life, I raced off to make the arrangements, telling everyone I passed about how God had used Esther to provide for my surgery. Everyone commented how they had never seen anyone so excited about having surgery. Well, this wasn't just any old surgery; I believe God had orchestrated every phase of this operation, and that Jon and Esther were willingly used as instruments in the hands of the Lord.

The surgery was scheduled for the next morning at eight a.m. I was so excited about the series of events that had gotten me this far that I had no fear, only complete and total faith that I was going to be cured. I had never experienced such joy! I felt like I was on top of the world! The last thing I remember before surgery was the anesthesiologist praying with me as he put me to sleep. When I awoke, the first thing I remember was the clock on the wall reading 10:15 a.m. Then I noticed that on either side of my bed were Jon and Esther, the dear angels the Lord had used to finance my surgery. Esther said they were supposed to leave the hospital that morning at eight a.m., but they were not going to leave until they knew that I was okay.

She went on to tell me that when they checked out, they were told they owed for vitamins and supplements that the hospital was sending home with them. She asked if I was going to also have a bill when I checked out of the hospital, and the receptionist said: "Yes. Everyone is sent home with vitamins." Esther patted my hand and said: "Don't worry about it. We left a check to cover the expenses. If it is more than they need, you just keep it."

Jon and Esther are indeed modern-day Good Samaritans, just like the story in Luke 10: 27-37. I was basically a stranger to these wonderful people, yet they made provision for my immediate need of surgery. Then they saw to it that all my expenses would be taken care of while I was in the hospital and beyond. What an awesome God we serve!

The surgery was a complete success. The doctor was able to remove the tumor, all the inflammatory tissue surrounding it, and do reconstructive surgery—all in just one surgery. Following surgery, I was required to take a vaccine made from the tumor that was removed from my body. I took the vaccine, orally, at first once a day for one week, then once a week for five weeks, and then only one time per month for the next seven months. I also took large quantities of vitamins, minerals, Omega 3's and enzymes.

I continued my diet of seventy percent fresh raw fruits and vegetables, juicing, and meals consisting of only thirty percent lean meat, organic rice, beans, nuts and dairy products.

In November 2007, I had a PET scan. The results came back clear. There was no sign of cancer in my body! I had won the battle!

I know the Lord is always with me; however, during the years I battled cancer, I felt His Presence more than ever before. Philippians 4:19 assures: *"God shall supply all your needs according to his riches in glory by Christ Jesus."* God, being always true to His Word, did indeed supply all my needs.

I believe God allowed me to get sick in order to strengthen my faith. Now, through this book, I pray that others going through similar health issues will also be encouraged and their faith in God's healing power strengthened. God designed us to be resilient. The psalmist says in Psalm 139:14: "I will praise You, for I am fearfully and wonderfully made…"

I pray the information provided in this book, will give you the courage and faith in God's *healing* power to give natural healing your first consideration. *Choose* to take control of your health. Natural treatments are *not* the easy way. You have to be involved with your diet and lifestyle on a *daily* basis. You can't just take a pill and expect to feel better immediately. However, your body will respond to healthy changes you make to your diet and lifestyle, *and* you will rapidly begin to see a reduction in your symptoms and experience the resilience and vitality God designed you with.

CHAPTER 2

HISTORY AND TESTIMONY
A DAY I WILL NEVER FORGET

I know God has been instrumental throughout my life, using my experiences, good and bad, to form and perfect me to become someone He can use to do His will. When I was diagnosed with cancer, I learned to put my faith in Him. During the process, He confirmed that He is the Great Physician and His creative hand is in natural healing.

On Wednesday evening, January 25, 2006—a day I will never forget—I discovered a lump in my breast. Instantly, I got the sickening feeling that I had breast cancer. My husband and I were uninsured at the time, which complicated the matter even further. I knew we did not have the financial means to seek treatment.

After spending a tearful and prayerful sleepless night, I contacted a local physician first thing the next morning.

I was amazed and delighted when he was able to schedule me immediately. Upon examination, he confirmed my suspicions, stating "the lump appears to be cancerous." He promptly sent me to a local hospital for a mammogram and ultrasound. The radiologist again confirmed my fears then sent me back to the physician to schedule an appointment with the surgeon.

The physician explained that I would be asked to sign papers allowing the surgeon to perform whatever type surgery he felt necessary and most effective to reduce the risk of the cancer spreading or recurring. The consent form would give the surgeon permission to do a total mastectomy rather than a simple lumpectomy, if he felt it would reduce my risk of developing breast cancer again in the future. My instant thought was "Of course, he will choose total mastectomy; the cancer can't recur if I don't have a breast." Then, after surgery, I would be required to have chemotherapy and radiation. I felt the physician was encouraging the most drastic treatment—a total mastectomy—followed by poisonous chemotherapy and radiation. This seemed extreme to me considering the lump was only the size of the tip of my thumb.

For the next several days, there was a continual gnawing in my stomach—a real hesitation about agreeing to such an extreme process without a second opinion. So, on Monday morning, I called and cancelled the appointment with the surgeon and contacted a specialist for a second opinion. He was supposedly the best in the area, so naturally he was booked up for weeks; but after pleading with his nurse, she amazingly worked me in by the end of the week.

Fortunately, my husband and I had the next few days to pray and contact friends and family members for moral support and encouragement. Two of our dearest colleagues and their wives, John and his wife Sharon and Jim and his wife Nellie, volunteered to loan us a total of $25,000 [interest free for five years] to help with medical expenses. God is so good! I know He is always with us and knows our every need even before we do. Matthew 6:8 (Amplified) says: *"Your Father (in heaven) knoweth what things ye have need of, before ye ask him."* Our prayers were answered; the financial concerns that were facing us had been lifted.

After researching the effects to one's body caused by the standard medical treatment for cancer, my long-standing confidence in the natural and alternative approaches to healing were reinforced. I couldn't even read about the devastating side effects of chemotherapy and radiation without bursting into tears. By the time I visited the surgeon, I was pretty well convinced that I would try an alternative form of treatment before undergoing extensive, mutilating surgery and subjecting my body to poisonous chemicals. However, I wanted to have a biopsy done to confirm that the lump was indeed cancerous and not just a cyst or some other form of tumor.

The surgeon told me about an insurance program offered by the state of Tennessee for women diagnosed with cancer. What a relief that was! I knew God had put the check in my spirit that I needed a second opinion, and He used my sister-in-law, Connie, to refer me to a physician who knew of this program—which relieved the stress and expense of going through such a devastating medical situation without insurance.

The biopsy was performed. Much to my amazement, it was completely painless; perhaps partially because I was on Cloud Nine. Whatever the diagnosis, the medical treatment would be covered, and my husband and I would not have to sell our home to pay for it. Another appointment was made to return in one week to receive the biopsy results.

Before returning for the results, I contacted the office of Dr. Dan Clark, the Naturopathic physician under whom I had studied. He had also treated me years before for migraine headaches. I felt confident he could diagnose the cause of my cancer through bio-energetic testing. This was the same way he had diagnosed the cause of my migraines years earlier. I believed he would be able to help me develop a natural treatment protocol to activate my body's natural responses—building up my immune system to detoxify my body, ultimately destroying the cancer cells that were overtaking my system. I knew my migraine headaches went away, and I believed my cancer would do the same.

I had suffered with migraine headaches from my early twenties well into my thirties: over fifteen years. Every month, I would start my period and within a day or two get a migraine headache that lasted for three days. I tried chiropractic treatment, medical treatment, and pharmaceutical drugs to relieve the pain. Nothing helped. The prescription drugs numbed the pain, but the headaches continued to come every month like clockwork.

I was introduced to Naturopathic medicine and bio-energetic testing one weekend while attending a medical conference. Without asking any health questions, a survey was performed using a probe that checked electrical impulses from the acupuncture points on my fingers and toes. These measurements apparently showed that my liver was toxic. I was told that I was probably having migraine headaches and had irregularity problems. Needless to say, I was amazed at the accuracy. I had suffered with both of these conditions for years. More than one physician said nothing could be done about the migraines with the exception of pain relieving drugs, and infrequent bowel movements are just normal for some people. I believe I was told that by the same physician who said: "All women are bitches, and there is nothing that can be done about it" when I asked him about my mood swings. No wonder I decided to study Naturopathic medicine!

I know a slow transit time through the intestines causes toxic waste to build up, enter the bloodstream, and affect our liver and various other organs of the body.[1] A toxic liver can cause migraine headaches; and research has proven that women who have two or fewer bowel movements per week have four times the risk of breast disease (benign or malignant) as women who have one or more bowel movements per day.[2]

The Naturopathic recommendation for treatment of my migraines was to take five homeopathic detoxifying remedies three times each day for the next three months.

1. *Constipation and Breast Cancer*, Saturday Evening Post, April 1982
2. Physicians Nicholas L. Petrakis and Eileen B. King of the University of California, writing in *Lancet*

I changed nothing in my diet or lifestyle—just put ten drops of each remedy under my tongue three times each day for the next three months. At the end of the first month, I did get the migraine, right on schedule, but it only lasted one day. That was exciting! The following month, I again got the migraine right on schedule, but it lasted only one hour. I couldn't believe it! By the third month, I didn't get a migraine at all! From that point to this day, I don't get migraine headaches! I believe strongly in Homeopathy and the natural healing approach to treatment for illness and disease. Now, years later, when confronted with another health issue, the natural, holistic approach was my choice.

When the biopsy results came back "positive," the surgeon recommended I speak to the oncologist so he could explain the treatment requirements. The oncologist told me that, after surgery, I would need to undergo seven weeks of daily radiation treatment followed by eight months of chemotherapy and be on numerous pharmaceutical drugs to reduce the chance of the cancer recurring. All this treatment was required, unless I agreed to a total mastectomy; and only then, if no cancer cells were detected in my lymph glands.

My medical background taught me that the lymph system is part of our body's protective mechanism. If undisturbed, the lymph is designed to overcome disease and, thereby, malignancy; however, it is significantly damaged and its effectiveness compromised by removal of the nodes.[3] Also, X-ray is dangerous and too much exposure will lead to cancer; chemotherapy is such a dangerous chemical that it destroys skin tissue if it comes into contact with it. Nurses are strictly warned against letting any of the chemical touch their skin or get onto their clothing. My review of some of the most commonly prescribed breast cancer drugs revealed their terrible side effects. For example, Herceptin can have serious effects such as heart damage, which may lead to heart failure. It can also affect the lungs, causing breathing problems. Avastin may cause problems with wound healing which could result in bleeding or infection; and Aromasin can cause vision problems, joint pain, headaches, high blood pressure, and a list of other miseries.

The risks of prolonged side effects from the standard medical approach to treatment were overwhelming. I knew that taking the natural treatment approach would activate my body's natural responses—building up my immune system and detoxify my body. All, without harsh side effects or the requirement to depend on pharmaceutical drugs for the rest of my life.

3. Cameron, Dr. Ewan and Pauling, Dr. Linus. *Alkalize For Health* http://www.alkalizeforhealth.net/rebounder.htm"

Therefore, on my return visit to the surgeon, I informed him I had decided to take an alternative approach to treating the cancer and believed God would guide and direct my path to recovery. The surgeon shook his head in disapproval and said he did not agree with my decision. He told me: "the only other patient I had that believed God would heal her was dead in six months." My feelings were that I would be a hypocrite if I just ignored all my training in natural healing, everything that I believed and preached to others, without even trying to allow my body to heal naturally. I knew that radiation and chemotherapy were poisons that would put added strain on my already weakened immune system, and both have been linked to the development of recurring cancer.

I walked out of the physician's office that day more determined than ever—feeling empowered and strengthened by my decision to prove the healing power of prayer—knowing that God would give me wisdom and guide and direct my path to healing. My firm belief in the healing power of God Almighty is assured in His words from Exodus 15:26: *"...For I am the Lord, who heals you."*

My faith was as Abraham's in Romans 4:19-21. ***"His faith did not weaken when he considered the impotence of his own body...no unbelief or distrust made him waver*** *concerning the promise of God. He grew strong and empowered by faith as he gave praise and glory to God, fully satisfied and assured that He was able and mighty to keep His word and do what He had promised."*

I also believe T. C. Fry was right when he said: "You cannot poison your body into health with drugs, chemo, or radiation. The holistic approach treats the whole animal, ignites the body's internal healing force and stimulates the body's natural abilities to heal itself. Health can only be achieved with healthful living."[4]

Natural treatment would not be covered by insurance. Thank God, our friends were moved to loan us the money we would need to pursue the natural approach to curing the cancer.

It seems a shame that insurance companies and our government willingly pay out hundreds of thousands of dollars for medical treatment only when recommended by allopathic (medical) physicians and only for standard treatment.

There is a plethora of evidence that natural and holistic methods of treatment are by far safer and frequently more effective. With the cost of cancer treatment increasing year after year and the dangerous side effects of cancer drugs,

---
4 http://www.alternativehealth.co.nz/cancer/index.htm

it seems our government and insurance companies would insist on offering patients alternative treatments for cancer therapy.

Dr. Whitaker says this about the treatment of cancer: "What is lost in the unemotional statistic of 500,000 cancer deaths per year is how those people died. In my opinion, conventional cancer therapy is so toxic and dehumanizing that I fear it far more than I fear death from cancer. We know that conventional therapy doesn't work—if it did, you would not fear cancer any more than you fear pneumonia. It is the utter lack of certainty as to the outcome of conventional treatment that virtually screams for more freedom of choice in the area of cancer therapy. Yet most so-called alternative therapies, regardless of potential or proven benefit, are outlawed, which forces patients to submit to the failures that we know don't work, because there's no other choice."[5]

Below is a story from an anonymous cancer patient. This serves as one example of how outrageous cancer treatment costs have become.

"Every three weeks, always on a Thursday afternoon, I amble on over to the cancer center for my IV treatment.

5. http://www.alternativehealth.co.nz/cancer/index.htm

(I also take Cytoxan, a chemo drug that comes in pill form, every day, plus a handful of other pills to help deal with the side effects and fringe benefits of being in cancer treatment—anxiety, high blood pressure, occasional depression, insomnia.)

The total bill for each treatment session at the cancer center is something north of $20,000. The annual cost of my cancer care is more than $300,000. That's three hundred thousand dollars a year. Almost, $30,000 a month to keep me alive.

Here's how the cost breaks down:

My bill from the Seattle Cancer Care Alliance (where I got my treatment until recently) for September 1, 2006, for three drugs - Herceptin, Avastin, and Zometa - was for $20,052.19.

The cost of the three drugs, listed as "drugs/ detail code," was $18,142.92. I asked at the pharmacy, and they told me that they charged me $6,254.95 for one dose of Herceptin, and an amazing $9,496.47 for one dose of Avastin.

In addition, SCCA charged me almost $2,000 to give me this one treatment.

I have included a chart from the National Cancer Institute which shows the rising cost of cancer treatment from 1963 through 2004—with an astonishing rise in cost from $1,300,000,000 to an unbelievable $72,100,000,000 in 2004. No wonder our nation's healthcare is at a crisis stage!

High cost of treating cancer

Since 1963, the cost of treating cancer has risen continuously, reaching $72.1 billion in 2004.

Cancer treatment spending, in billions:
- 1963: $1.3
- 1972:
- 1980:
- 1985: $13.1
- 1990:
- 1995: $27.5
- 2004: $72.1

Average Medicare payments*, per individual:
Ovary	$36,800
Esophagus	30,500
Pancreas	26,600
Kidney	25,300
Lung	24,700
Colorectal	24,200
Lymphoma	21,500
Cervix	20,100
Head/neck	18,000
Leukemia	18,000

Percentage of all new cancers, 1998:
- Prostate: 16.8%
- Breast: 15.9
- Lung: 12.7
- Colorectal: 10.7
- Other: 43.9

*In first year following diagnosis, in 2004 dollars

SOURCE: National Cancer Institute   AP

I was not sure what the cost would be to cure cancer naturally, but I did know it would cost considerably less than the standard medical treatment. My philosophy was that it would be better to restore my body to health through natural means. I didn't believe that poisoning my body with chemotherapy drugs or burning it with radiation was the way back to health.

I so strongly believed this treatment choice was the right one for me, a win-win decision, that I had no fear. I believed as Paul did in his letter to the Philippians [1:21]: ***"For to me, to live is Christ, and to die is gain."*** I knew I would rather trust in God than in man. If in the process I was healed, what a wonderful testimony I would have! If I died, I would spend eternity with my Heavenly Father! See, I could not lose!

I have laced this book with many encouraging quotes and Scripture after Scripture assuring of God's love and compassion. These and many more messages inspired me and strengthened me to continue when no improvement in my condition was obvious.

Over one hundred years ago, Thomas Edison (1847-1931) said: "The doctor of the future will give no medicine, but will interest her or his patients in the care of the human frame, in a proper diet, and in the cause and prevention of disease" and "The doctor of the future will no longer treat the human frame with drugs, but rather will cure and prevent disease with nutrition.[5]" Jethro Kloss said: "God, in His infinite wisdom, neglected nothing and if we would eat our food without trying to improve, change or refine it, thereby destroying its life-giving elements, it would meet all requirements of the body.[6]"

---

5. http://www.quotationspage.com/quotes/Thomas_A._Edison/
6. Kloss, Jethro. *Back to Eden.* 1939

Edison and Kloss knew that disease is caused by the effects of an improper diet and stress and, therefore, can be cured if we use what God has created in its natural form and not exist entirely on foods robbed of their life-giving elements and packed with artificial ingredients, preservatives, food coloring, and other additives.

This is the story about what I did and did not do during the course of the next two years to help restore my body to health and defeat the cancer the natural way. I wrote this book because the Word of God commands us to tell of our blessings and miracles so that others will be encouraged and their faith will be increased.

Matthew 5:16 tells us: ***"Let your light so shine before men, that they may see your good works and glorify your Father in heaven."***

Hopefully, through this book I will help others understand how our bodies are designed and what our bodies need to be healthy and to heal. Then, putting your faith and trust in God and through prayer and praise, lay your cares upon Jesus, do your part to give your body the nutrition it needs to regain health, and I believe you too will experience healing miracles. The scripture Psalm 139:14 says it so well, ***"I praise you because I am fearfully and wonderfully made; your works are wonderful, I know that full well."***

"The secret of health for both mind and body is not to mourn for the past, not to worry about the future, or not to anticipate troubles, but to live the present moment wisely and earnestly."

Gautama Buddha

CHAPTER 3

HEALING PRAYERS

My initial treatment started with intensive prayers for healing and asking God to lead my research and divulge whatever method was necessary to heal my body of cancer. I immediately began praising God for my healing and for giving me the opportunity to prove He is the Great Physician. Mark 11:24 ***"Therefore I say unto you, What things soever ye desire, when ye pray, believe that ye receive them, and ye shall have them."*** Healing Prayers are for all those who long for the healing power of our Lord and Savior. These prayers are offered in faith and hope that, we might all experience healing of body, mind and spirit in every aspect of our lives.

Our desire for healing, or wholeness, is directly related to our faith in God and to our openness to the love of the Holy Spirit. If we truly believe in God's power to heal and in His deep love for us, God will guide us with His infinite wisdom in every situation and circumstance. As we turn our needs over to God in prayer, healing can and will occur.

We tend to think of 'healing' only in a physical sense. But healing can and does have a much broader significance in our lives. The words 'health', 'healing', 'holiness', and 'wholeness' are all derived from the same root word, 'hal', which means whole or unhurt. True healing involves not only the physical but also the mental, emotional, and spiritual aspects of our lives.

There is no "right" or "best" way to pray for healing, what is most important is not how we pray, but only that we pray. When we pray, God is there for us; He is listening to our prayers and touching our lives with His healing and love.

Matthew 7:7 *"Ask, and it shall be given you; seek, and ye shall find; knock, and it shall be opened unto you: For every one that asketh receiveth; and he that seeketh findeth; and to him that knocketh it shall be opened."*

2 Kings 20:5 *"Thus saith the LORD, the God of David thy father, I have heard thy prayer, I have seen thy tears: behold, I will heal thee."*

Mark 9:23 *"Jesus said unto him, If thou canst believe, all things are possible to him that believeth."*

Matthew 8:13 *"...As thou hast believed, so be it done unto thee."*

1 Thessalonians 5:17 *"Pray without ceasing."*

Isaiah 41:10 *"...Do not be afraid, for I am with you; stop being anxious and watchful, for I am your God. I give you strength, I bring you help, I uphold you with my victorious right hand."*

ST. FRANCIS' PRAYER

Lord, make me an instrument of Your peace.
Where there is hatred, let me sow love,
Where there is injury, pardon.
Where there is discord, union.
Where there is doubt, faith.
Where there is despair, hope.
Where there is darkness, light.
And where there is sadness, joy.
O Master, grant that I may not so much seek
to be consoled, as to console;
to be understood, as to understand;
to be loved, as to love;
for it is in giving that we receive.
It is in pardoning that we are pardoned.
And it is in dying that we are born to eternal life.

James 1:5

"If any of you lack wisdom, let him ask of God,
that giveth to all men liberally,
and upbraideth not;
and it shall be given him."

CHAPTER 4

TREATMENT DECISIONS

The treatment method I chose would require a monthly trip to see Dr. Jonathan Clark in Melbourne, Florida. At his clinic, I would be tested using the Computron, a bio-energetic device that checks acupressure points (meridians) throughout the body and gives readings on each organ system. "Because the meridians influence every cell in the body and pass through every organ and organ system, acupuncture (meridians) provides the health practitioners with an accurate and noninvasive means of determining health deficiencies as well as a method of reestablishing balance."[1] Using this technology, one can determine the effectiveness of various nutrients, remedies, vitamins, and minerals on balancing and bringing the organ system back into harmony.

1 *William Michael Cargile, B.S., D.C., F.I.A.C.A., Chairman of Research for the American Association of Acupuncture and Oriental Medicine*

I quickly found out:

vitamins, minerals, and other natural substances can be as expensive as pharmaceutical drugs because something natural is touted as being helpful for a particular condition does not mean it will work effectively for everyone. Combining nutritional supplements can be as dangerous as combining pharmaceutical drugs taking the wrong combination of supplements wastes precious time and money.

The technology to check the effectiveness of drugs and natural remedies has been available to the medical profession and recognized as accurate by the Food and Drug Administration for many years. I believe this technology should be required to be used by every physician, pharmacist, dietician, and health food store in the world before they recommend or prescribe anything to their patients. However, our physicians continue to prescribe drugs without knowing what side effects they will have on their patients or if they will even be effective for the condition for which they are being prescribed.

Have you ever heard the saying "What you don't know won't hurt you?" That cannot be farther from the truth! What you don't know about staying healthy *CAN* keep you ill or kill you!

Our physicians should stop "practicing" and

experimenting on us and start prescribing only the supplements and products that would actually help heal us, without causing dangerous side effects. It upsets me when someone tells me their physician has prescribed drug after drug, instructing them to stop taking them if they have any of the dozens of potential side effects that the literature mentions. Patients are mere guinea pigs when it comes to prescription drugs. This haphazard approach to treating illness and disease could be eliminated with technology that has already been proven.

There is an abundance of documented information regarding the limitations and abuse of our modern medical establishment, which also bolstered my decision to take the natural approach to healing. Listed below are quotes from outspoken medical professionals concerning the state of our healthcare system and our out-of-control pharmaceutical costs? The United States spends more on healthcare and pharmaceutical drugs than any other nation in the world, and according to Forbes statistics, the United States is not even listed in the top ten healthiest countries.

Research done by Robert I. Bender, M.D., FAAFP, found that from 1960 to 1980, prescription drug sales were fairly steady as a percentage of the U.S. gross domestic product; but from 1980 to 2000, they tripled, and according to the Retail Drug Monitor (IMS): "Global pharmaceutical sales through retail pharmacies increased 5% in just one year between November 2005 and November 2006, standing now at 386.23 billion per year."[2]

In 2002, the combined profits for the ten drug companies on the Fortune 500 list was 35.9 billion dollars. All the other 490 businesses put together brought in only 33.7 billion dollars. This means that the top ten drug companies made more profit than all the other Fortune 500 companies put together.[3]

According to Dr. Mercola, America has the best system in the entire world for treating acute surgical emergencies. However; beyond that, the system is an unmitigated failure at treating chronic illness.[4]

When compared to other developed countries, the United States falls behind in terms of life expectancy. It is not among the top ten in the world and, in fact, is among those countries of the world at the lower end of the scale. The U.S. life expectancy level is close to that of Cuba.[5]

2. Heath Ledger Legacy: *Prescription Drugs a Silent Killer*. Sept.29, 2008
3. Angell, Marcia. *Excess in the pharmaceutical industry*. CMAJ Dec 7, 2004;
4. Dr. Mercola. *US Health System Most Expensive in the World*. Jan 2, 2008
5. *Epidemiology And Today's Deadliest Diseases*. http://www.videojug.com/interview/epidemiology-and-todays-deadliest-diseases-2

According to the Journal of the American Medical Association (JAMA), prescription drugs are now the fourth leading medical cause of death in the U.S. and Canada, behind only cancer, heart disease and stroke which "are facilitated largely by physician ignorance of foundational concepts of nutritional physiology."[6]

According to William J. Kassler, past President of the AMSA, "the teaching of nutrition in most U.S. medical schools is inadequate. Education has traditionally focused on the principles of acute episodic health-care delivery, overlooking the concepts and application of nutrition and preventive medicine. Nutrition is not well taught, if taught at all, in most medical schools".[7]

A recent study titled Nutrition Education in US Medical Schools, performed by the University of North Carolina, learned that almost all schools now require exposure to nutrition; however, only about a quarter offered the recommended 25 hours of instruction and only a quarter of the schools managed to have a single course dedicated to the topic.[8]

6. *4th Leading Cause of Death in U.S. Prescription Drugs.* 12/9/09 Drug Alert. http://www.the7thfire.com/health_and_nutrition/Prescription_drugs_"_deaths.htm.
7. Kassler, William J., AMSA National President, *Testimony of the American Medical Studen Assoviation: Nutrition Eduation in the Undergraduate Medical Curriculum,* page 121, January 14, 1985
8. DiNapoli, Marianne, *Nutrition – a gap in medical education,* Sep. 16, 2010

It is because American medical doctors continue to focus on acute episodic health-care delivery and overlooking the concepts and application of nutrition and preventive medicine. That the physical health of Americans continues to deteriorate, with increasing numbers of chronically ill people with no hope of recovery and a life spent in a suspended state of ill health and dependence on pharmaceutical drugs, which empties their pocket books and destroys any hope of restoration.

Each year, prescription drugs cause seriousreactions and permanent disability for over 2.2 million people. More people are killed by prescription drugs each year than were killed in the entire Vietnam War.[9]

An article by Drs. Holland and DeGruy suggests that as many as ten percent of hospital admissions may be attributable to prescription drug-induced disorders.[10]

Two facts many people do not realize are:

1) prescription drugs can be as dangerous as street drugs.
2) "the vast majority of drugs—more than 90 percent—only work in 30% to 50% of the people."

---

9. Bender, Robert I, M.D., FAAFP. *The Pharmaceutical "Business with Disease"* September 29, 2008
10. Holland and DeGruy. *American Academy of Family Physician.* June 1998

According to Dr. Allen Roses, the worldwide vice president of GlaxoSmithKline. "Cancer drugs only work 25% of the time, Alzheimer's drugs work 30% of the time, and many others only 50% of the time."[11] On average, fifty-one percent of drugs approved by the Food and Drug Administration (FDA) have serious adverse side effects that are not detected prior to their approval for public use. This is why most pharmaceuticals actually contribute to hospitalization, permanent disabilities, disease, illness, and death. The "Father of Medicine," Hippocrates is well-known for saying "as far as disease, help or at least do no harm." Unfortunately, it appears that the pharmaceutical industry is more focused on making a profit than curing disease.[12]

The pharmaceutical industry spends more than twice as much on advertising and administration as they spend on research. Since 1990, drug rates have gone up 500%.

Advertisements on television, radio, and in national publications are constantly promoting everything from drugs for serious to mild ailments. This encourages people to diagnose their own condition and request drugs from their physician.

11. Connor, Steve. Glaxo Chief: *Our Drugs Do Not Work on Most Patients, Common Dreams*. December 8, 2003
12. Cohen, Jay, M.D. *Campaign for Truth, The Case Against the Drug Companies*. February 2002

Advertisements on television, radio, and in national publications are constantly promoting everything from drugs for serious to mild ailments. This encourages people to diagnose their own condition and request drugs from their physician.

Peter R. Breggin, M.D., the former consultant at the National Institute of Mental Health, and author of the book *Medical Madness,* stated: "The population of North America is one of the most heavily medicated in the world," and that "the profitable pharmaceutical industry has created a disturbingly legal drug addicted society."[13]

If I had chosen the standard medical treatment and survived, I would have always wondered if I survived not because of the drugs and surgery but in spite of them.

As I searched for natural cures for cancer, these promises from God's Word encouraged me to continue seeking. According to James 1:5: *"If any of you lack wisdom, let him ask of God, that giveth to all men liberally, and upbraideth not; and it shall be given him."* Also in Matthew 7:7: *"Ask, and it shall be given you; seek, and ye shall find; knock, and it shall be opened unto you."*

---

13 Breggin, Peter R., MD. *Medical Madness.* July 2008

I found over three hundred proven cures for cancer described in-depth during my research, along with a plethora of testimonials from common people that had opted out of standard medical treatments and been healed of not only cancer but a multitude of other illnesses. My prayer was that God would guide me to what my body needed in order to be restored to health, and that He give me faith to stand firm in His healing power. I also prayed for wisdom for the Naturopathic physician treating me.

On my first visit to the Naturopathic physician, he warned me to stay away from negative people. It is crucial that one's mind and spirit remain positive and uplifted. Heed the Apostle Paul's instructions in Philippians 4:8: *"Finally, brethren, whatsoever things are true, whatsoever things are honest, whatsoever things are just, whatsoever things are pure, whatsoever things are lovely, whatsoever things are of good report; if there be any virtue, and if there be any praise, think on these things."*

A positive mental attitude and faith in the healing power of God empowers your body and stimulates the healing process.

Philippians 4:7

"And the peace of God, which passeth all understanding, shall keep your hearts and minds through Christ Jesus."

CHAPTER 5

SKEPTICISM

The one thing I was not prepared for was the skepticism some people have about the treatment option I chose. When I was warned by my Naturopathic physician to stay away from negative people, I did not realize it would be some of those so closes to me. The Bible instructs in 2 Corinthians 6:14-15: *"Do not be unequally yoked together with unbelievers.... what part has a believer with an unbeliever?"*

To stand firm in my belief in God's healing power, it was essential to avoid those whose belief was inconsistent with my faith. For all their well-intended concern, the roughest part of the next two years of my life was by far the agony I felt because of others' negative opinions and disbelief in what I was doing.

They believed I had lost my mind and was committing suicide because I opted out of what the so-called medical professionals told me was my only option.

Some, were willing to help in any way possible when they first heard of my diagnosis. Offering to stay with me, take me to the doctor's office, clean my house, or prepare meals for me—whatever I needed during the devastating treatment. However, when I told them I was going to put my faith in God and trust that everything I had learned in my medical training was factual, their concern turned to fear and skepticism. To them, my education was irrelevant. It reminded me of the story in Mark 6:4: "But Jesus said to them, *"A prophet is not without honor except in his own country, among his own relatives, and in his own house."* I realized there was nothing I could say to give others confidence in my decision. I prayed daily as the Apostle Paul in Philippians 4:7: *"(That) the peace of God, which passeth all understanding, shall keep (their) hearts and minds through Christ Jesus."* Only God could give them peace because they could not understand my faith or my commitment to natural healing.

I had many conversations with God about how it was going to look, if I didn't recover from this illness. I had announced to the world that my faith and trust was in God's miraculous healing power and my belief that He designed our bodies to heal themselves of disease if given the proper nutrition.

I did everything within my power to restore my body to health and remained focused and confident, reciting constantly:

I am healed in the name of Jesus,
Cancer has no hold on me.

The one family member that actually encouraged my decision to battle the cancer through natural means as opposed to the standard medical approach was Aunt Nancy, my Dad's youngest sister. She lost her husband a few years earlier, after a long and difficult struggle with cancer. They followed the doctor's recommendations to the letter—suffering through countless hours of chemotherapy, radiation, and other treatments that destroyed my uncle's quality of life and, in the end, only prolonged his agony.

My family and I had always been very close; however, we were at odds over my choice to take control of my own health and, in essence, my own life. It was those who believed in the healing power of prayer and our Lord and Savior's promises that were my strength during this difficult struggle. ***"For whoever does the things God wills is My brother and sister and mother!"*** [Mark 3:35, Amplified]

I made a point to tell everyone I met, any time I was out shopping, walking, et cetera, that I was battling breast cancer naturally, with prayer and diet. It seemed a good opportunity to minister to others. Everyone always said: "Good luck! We will pray for you." One day, I mentioned to someone that everyone who didn't know me very well was rooting for me, while my family thought I was crazy. Their response was a revelation. They said: "That's because we don't love you." I finally realized that my family wasn't against me—they just didn't understand and were afraid for me!

In hindsight, I realize that in many ways the skepticism and lack of faith in natural healing of some of those so close to me had actually forced me to think and speak positively at all times. I knew if I ever said anything negative they would be even more concerned. Therefore, I always said I was doing well! Feeling great! I had to step out of the limitations of my childhood teachings and take the Word of God literally, believing Hebrews 13:8: ***Jesus Christ the same yesterday, and today, and forever.*** My life depended on God working miraculously, and He did!

Chapter 5

What I Did and Why I Did It

My daily routine became extremely regimented. In order to focus totally on getting well, I gave up my job. I actually made a checklist to ensure that I didn't forget any part of the required program throughout the day.

Following is a list of the daily nutrition I took [the rest and exercise protocol I designed from my extensive research is covered in a following section]. Each item is listed with a brief description of its content, if applicable, and explanation of its importance in the overall program. In the following sections, I will elaborate on what I feel are the most important topics and the effect each has on one's body in the healing process.

This quote from a well-known source helped to confirm that my decision to go natural was the right one:

"AS A RETIRED PHYSICIAN, I CAN HONESTLY SAY THAT UNLESS YOU ARE IN A SERIOUS ACCIDENT, YOUR BEST CHANCE OF LIVING TO A RIPE OLD AGE IS TO AVOID DOCTORS AND HOSPITALS AND LEARN NUTRITION, HERBAL MEDICINE, AND OTHER FORMS OF NATURAL MEDICINE.

Almost all drugs are toxic and are designed only to treat symptoms and not to cure anyone. Most surgery is unnecessary. In short, our mainstream medical system is hopelessly inept and/or corrupt.

THE TREATMENT OF DEGENERATIVE DISEASES AND CANCER IS A NATIONAL SCANDAL.

The sooner you learn this, the better off you will be."[1]

1. Greenberg, Allen, Dr. *Prevention*, 12/24/2002

CHAPTER 7

DAILY REGIMEN

First thing each morning, prepare 8 ounces of warm purified water with the juice from ½ of a freshly squeezed lemon, than add a generous shake of cayenne pepper—This helps to balance the body's pH.

Drink this before taking anything else.

• Prepare vegetable juice for the day—Raw vegetable juice provides essential nutrients, enzymes and keeps the bodies pH balanced.

• Prepare green tea. I would drink up to 6 cups each day. Green Tea Polyphenols (GTP), particularly EGCG or EGCg (epigallocatechin gallate) not only inhibit an enzyme required for cancer cell growth, but also kills cancer cells with no ill effect on healthy cells.[1]

Researchers from the University of Kansas determined that EGCG is twice as powerful as resveratrol, which itself is known to kill cancer cells.[2]

- Herbs such as fresh parsley, cilantro and garlic were added to my vegetable juice and daily meals. Hebrews 6:7: **"For the soil which has drunk the rain that repeatedly falls upon it and produces vegetation useful to those for whose benefit it is cultivated partakes of a blessing from God."**

- One-half [½] hour after drinking lemon water, take four [4] ounces freshly juiced wheat grass or alfalfa sprouts – this stimulates balancing of neuro-endocrine system and activates T and B cells

- Rebounding, ten [10] minutes, three [3] to four [4] times each day—Rebounding on a mini-trampoline improves breathing patterns, stimulates lymphatic drainage, and improves cellular balance

- Wobenzyme, forty-five [45] minutes before each meal—enzymes taken before meals work at the cellular level to improve metabolism

1. Purdue University, cancertutorial.com
2. University of Kansas study, 1997

- Stretching/breathing exercise/walking, forty- five [45] minutes—improves lymph drainage and increases breathing, which stimulates oxygen uptake thereby reducing muscle tension and mental stress

- Eight [8] ounces purified water—hydration is vitally important to detoxification and proper organ function

- Dry skin brushing—cleans skin and circulates and cleanses the lymph—aiding in the elimination process. Use a natural brush on all areas of the skin [except face and any sensitive areas] with long strokes toward the heart prior to shower or bath. The brush and skin are both dry when brushing is performed.

- Breakfast—organic oatmeal or fruit with nuts, organic naturally-sweetened yogurt or veggie omelet.

- Goat's milk—eight [8]—sixteen [16] ounces, this is one of the best food medicines for rebuilding the brain, nervous system, and mental faculties. It also works to regenerate the cells of the body.

- Vitamins that need to be taken with food (multi-vitamins, multi-minerals, omega-3, Hepasil DTX).

- Homeopathic remedies, one [1] hour after meals—helps in detoxification

- Eight [8]—sixteen [16] ounces of vegetable juice – provides digestive enzymes, nutrition, and balances pH

- Lunch—salad, veggie wrap, or homemade vegetable broth soup

- Four [4] ounces Aloe Vera juice—helps activate white blood cells and promotes growth of non-cancerous cells. The National Cancer Institute has included Aloe Vera in their recommendations for increased testing because of its apparent cancer-fighting properties. Leviticus 17:11: "For the life of the flesh is in the blood…"

- Vitamins that need to be taken with food.

- Breathing exercises/walking outdoors for one [1] hour. Walking improves breathing patterns, stimulates lymphatic drainage, and improves cellular balance. The best time to receive adequate sun exposure is between 11:00 a.m. and 2:00 p.m. It is recommended to get at least ten [10] minutes of direct exposure on your arms and face at least three [3] times a week to maintain proper vitamin D levels

- Eight [8] ounces of water—to maintain hydration

- Homeopathic remedies, one [1] hour after meals—detoxification

- One [1] ounce flaxseed oil and four [4] ounces cottage cheese—Dr. Johanna Budwig's cancer diet treats patients with a mixture of flax oil and quark (a kind of cottage cheese). The omega-3 essential oil available from flax oil and ground flax seed is a proven cancer fighter and is required for proper kidney function

- Rest and Christian meditation (one hour) between 3 and 5 p.m.

- Dinner—fish or lean meat, whole grain rice and fresh, raw vegetables and herbs. Exodus 12:8: **"And they shall eat the flesh in that night, roast with fire, and unleavened bread; and with bitter herbs they shall eat it."**

- Cold water, ocean fish contains Docosahexanoic acid (DHA), an omega-3 fatty acid which has been shown to reduce the size of tumors

- Vitamins that need to be taken with food

- Homeopathic remedies, one [1] hour after meals, detoxification

- Breathing exercise/Rebounder, ten [10] minutes—lymph drainage

- One [1] ounce flaxseed oil and four [4] ounces cottage cheese—Dr. Budwig's cancer cure remedy. Flaxseed oil is rich in omega-3

- Sleep at least eight [8] hours, preferably between 9 p.m. and 6 a.m.

CHAPTER 8

HOMEOPATHIC REMEDIES

I took each of these items at some time during my treatment; however, my nutrition was adjusted as my condition improved:

Mammory plex—stimulates normal mammary function and drainage of breast lymphatics

Metalogin—heavy metal detoxification; dental amalgam, and other metals' detoxification

Inflammation—reduces inflammation and swelling

Systemic Detox—stimulation of the lymph and spleen, liver, and blood

Additox—insecticide detoxifier; stimulates release of insecticides into lymphatics

Romans 14:2

"For one believeth that he may eat all things: another, who is weak, eateth herbs."

CHAPTER 9

BOTANICAL HERBS

Artemesioplex—contains wormwood which has a cleansing effect on the stomach, liver, and intestine.

Cilantro—proven to help combat cancer—contains caffeic acid and chlorogenic acid antioxidants—two acids that trap the free radicals. Eating just a teaspoon of fresh cilantro every day cuts the risk of cancer.[1]

Gerplex II—cleanses the lymphatic glands and purifies the blood.

Vermaplex—fortifies the colon and encourages parasite expulsion.

[1]. Whatley, T., *Hydrogen Sulf 3X The Undeniable Benefits of Cilantro*, Whitney Worden, Dec. 29, 2008

Scrofularoplex—stimulates lymphatic drainage of glandular swelling and congestion in chronic swollen lymph nodes and tenderness in the breast.

Burdock—includes chelidonium containing ten (10) alkaloids which retard tumor growth and a recently identified chemical (arctigenin) which acts as an inhibitor of tumor growth.[2]

Trifoloplex—stimulates drainage of breast lymphatics and spleen, also a lymphatic cleanser and endocrine balancer.

---

2. *Natural Cancer Treatment.* 10/14/2008

CHAPTER 10

Drainage

Lymph III—helps drain enlarged lymph glands, reduces exhaustion, and emaciation.

Hydrate I—helps with water absorption.

Liver Tonic III—stimulates liver detoxification from chemical toxicity.

Nutritional Support—supplements providing macro and micro nutrients to aid immune system and metabolic function.

HypoScorbate—Vitamin C has been found to be beneficial for strengthening the immune system, stress, depression, and cancer prevention.

Natura 401—601—stimulates lymph drainage.

Selenium EC—a component in antioxidant enzymes—it helps prevent DNA damage, boosts immune function, and inhibits growth of blood vessels upon which tumors are dependent and induces cancer cells to self-destruct. Germanium - a trace element (mineral) which promotes cell oxygen absorption.

Bio Mer Detox—heavy metal detoxification product which helps remove mercury from the body.

CoQ10—plays a key role in producing energy in the mitochondria, the part of a cell responsible for the production of energy in the form of ATP.

Mega Antioxidants—antioxidants act as "free radical scavengers" hence preventing or repairing damage done by free radicals.

Hepasil DTX—Stimulates detox of liver

Bio Green—elimination of body wastes and toxins, protection from harmful environmental pollution, aids in proper cellular metabolism, improved resistance to stress, memory enhancer, and increases energy levels.

Chlorella—contains vitamin C and carotenoids, antioxidant compounds that block the action of free radicals, activated oxygen molecules that can damage cells. Chlorella also contains high concentrations of B-complex vitamins. It strengthens the immune system and increases the level of albumin in the body, protecting against diseases such as cancer through its ability to cleanse the body of toxins and heavy metals.

Spirulina—is richly supplied with the blue pigment phycocyanim, an antigen shown to inhibit cancer- colony formation.

Sea Salt—contains vitamins, minerals, macro-minerals, trace minerals, phytonutrients, and all the essential amino acids.

Waiora Natural Cellular Defense—natural volcanic minerals work at the cellular level, trapping heavy metals and toxins. Because it is a negatively charged mineral, it acts as a magnet, drawing toxins—capturing and removing them from the body.[1]

---

1. Products and information provided by BIOActive Nutritional, Inc & Better Health & Wellness Center

CHAPTER 11

FOODS AND THEIR HEALTH BENEFITS

The following food chart is an easy reference guide to the health benefits of many common foods. It was e-mailed to me by my dear friend, Antoinette Sequeira, with instructions to send it to everyone I know. I can think of no better way to share this helpful and informative list than by including it in this book.

"Thank you" to whoever compiled this wonderful chart.

Apples	Protect your heart	Prevent constipation	Block diarrhea	Improve lung capacity	Cushion joints
Apricots	Combat cancer	Control blood pressure	Save eyesight	Shield against Alzheimer's	Slow aging
Artichokes	Aid digestion	Lower cholesterol	Protect your heart	Stabilize blood sugar	Guard against liver disease
Avocados	Battle diabetes	Lower cholesterol	Help stop strokes	Control blood pressure	Smoothe skin

Bananas	Protect your heart	Quiet coughs	Strengthen bones	Control blood pressure	Block diarrhea
Beans	Prevent constipation	Help hemorrhoids	Lower cholesterol	Combat cancer	Stabilize blood sugar
Beets	Control blood pressure	Combat cancer	Strengthen bones	Protect your heart	Aid weight loss
Blueberries	Combat cancer	Protect your heart	Stabilize blood sugar	Boost memory	Prevent constipation
Broccoli	Strengthen bones	Save eyesight	Combat cancer	Protect your heart	Control blood pressure
Cabbage	Combat cancer	Prevent constipation	Promote weight loss	Protect your heart	Help hemorrhoids
Cantaloupe	Saves eyesight	Controls blood pressure	Lowers cholesterol	Combats cancer	Supports immune system
Carrots	Save eyesight	Protect your heart	Prevent constipation	Combat cancer	Promote weight loss
Cauliflower	Protects against prostate cancer	Combats breast cancer	Strengthen bones	Banishes bruises	Guards against heart diasease
Cherries	Protect your heart	Combat cancer	End insomnia	Slow aging	Shield against Alzheimer's

Chestnuts	Promote weight loss	Protect your heart	Lower cholesterol	Combat cancer	Control blood pressure
Chili Peppers	Aids digestion	Soothe sore throat	Clear sinuses	Combat cancer	Boost immune system
Figs	Promote weight loss	Help stop strokes	Lower cholesterol	Combat cancer	Control blood pressure
Cold Water Ocean Fish	Lowers blood pressure & blood triglycerides	Boost memory Lowers Alzheimer's risk & depression	Omega-3 fatty acids protect your heart	Reduce inflammation rheumatoid arthritis gout psoriasis	Support immune system lower risk of cancer
Flax	Aids digestion	Battles diabetes	Protect your heart	Improves mental health	Boost immune system
Garlic	Lowers cholesterol	Controls blood pressure	Combats cancer	Kills bacteria	Fights Fungus
Grapefruit	Protects against heart attacks	Promote weight loss	Help stop strokes	Combats prostate cancer	Lowers cholesterol
Grapes	Save eyesight	Conquer kidney stones	Combat cancer	Enhance blood flow	Protect your heart
Green Tea	Combats cancer	Protects your heart	Helps stop strokes	Promotes weight loss	Kills bacteria

93

Honey	Heals wounds	Aids digestion	Guards against ulcers	Increases energy	Fights allergies
Lemons	Combats cancer	Protect your heart	Controls blood pressure	Smoothe skin	Stop scurvy
Limes	Combat cancer	Protect your heart	Control blood pressure	Smoothe skin	Stop scurvy
Mangoes	Combat cancer	Boost memory	Regulate thyroid	Aid digestion	Shield against Alzheimer's
Mushrooms	Control blood pressure	Lower cholesterol	Kill bacteria	Combat cancer	Strengthen bones
Oats	Lower cholesterol	Combat cancer	Battle diabetes	Prevent constipation	Smoothe skin
Olive Oil	Protects your heart	Promotes weight loss	Combat cancer	Battles diabetes	Smoothes skin
Onions	Reduce risk of heart attack	Combat cancer	Kill bacteria	Lower cholesterol	Fights fungus
Oranges	Support immune sytems	Combat cancer	Protect your heart	Strengthen respiration	Blood clot inhibiting properties
Peaches	Prevent constipation	Combat cancer	Helps stop strokes	Aids digestion	Help hemorrhoids

94

Peanuts	Protect your heart	Promote weight loss	Combat prostate cancer	Lowers cholesterol	Reduces diverticulitis
Pineapple	Strengthen bones	Relieves colds	Aids digestion	Dissolves warts	Blocks diarrhea
Prunes	Slows aging process	Prevent constipation	Boost memory	Lowers cholesterol	Protect your heart
Rice	Protects your heart	Battles diabetes	Conquers kidney stones	Combat cancer	Helps stop strokes
Strawberries	Combat cancer	Protects your heart	Boost memory	Calm stress	Protect cells from free radicals
Sweet Potatoes	Save eyesight	Lift mood	Combat cancer	Strengthen bones	Blood sugar regulator lowers insulin resistance
Tomatoes	Protect prostate	Combat cancer	Lowers cholesterol	Protects your heart	Contain Lycopenea powerful antioxidant
Walnu's	Lowers cholesterol	Combat cancer	Boost memory	Lift mood	Protects against heart disease
Water	Promotes weight loss	Combats cancer	Conquers kidney stones	Smoothes skin	Prevent constipation

Watermelon	Protects prostate	Promotes weight loss	Lowers cholesterol	Helps stop strokes	Control blood pressure
Wheat Germ	Combats colon cancer	Prevent constipation	Lowers cholesterol	Helps stop strokes	Aids digestion
Wheat Bran	Combats colon cancer	Prevent constipation	Lowers cholesterol	Helps stop strokes	Aids digestion
Yogurt	Guards against ulcers	Strengthen bones	Lowers cholesterol	Supports immune systems	Aids digestion

Deuteronomy 5:33

Ye shall **walk** *in all the ways which the LORD your God hath* **commanded** *you, that ye may live, and that it may be* **well** *with you, and that ye may prolong your days in the land which ye shall possess.*

CHAPTER 12

Understanding Your Body

WITH SPIRITUAL AND TWENTY-FIRST CENTURY REFERENCES

I believe the more a person understands about how their body works, the more inclined they will be to make the healthy choices necessary to enhance both the quantity and quality of their life! It's been said "the greatest wealth is health...!" What good is all the money in the world if a person is incapable of enjoying it in good health?

I once heard a comedian say: "If I knew I was going to live so long, I would have taken better care of myself." Of course, that joke aroused a great deal of laughter. In reality, that sentiment needs to be taken very seriously. We only get one life and one body! If we abuse that body, we will suffer in our lifetime.

In 1 Corinthians 6:19-20, the Bible tells us: ***"... Know ye not that your body is the temple of the Holy Ghost*** *which is in you, which ye have of God, and ye are not your own? For you were bought at a price; therefore glorify God in your body, and in your spirit, which are God's."* We are the caretakers of the temple of the Holy Ghost. In that capacity, we are required to live wise and healthy lives.

If we take our guidance from the Word of God for our mental, physical, and spiritual living, we enjoy long and healthy lives. Ephesians 6:3 *"That it may be well with thee, and thou mayest live long on the earth."* We must not, however, expect that we will live forever. Our goal should be to remain healthy as long as we are alive.

The Word of God specifically states in these beautiful verses in Ecclesiastes 3:1-8 *"There is an appointed time for everything and that each of us has a time to die:*

> *There is a time for everything,*
> *and a season for every activity under heaven:*
> *a time to be born and a time to die,*
> *a time to plant and a time to uproot,*
> *a time to kill and a time to heal,*
> *a time to tear down and a time to build,*
> *a time to weep and a time to laugh,*
> *a time to mourn and a time to dance,*

a time to scatter stones and a time to gather them,
a time to embrace and a time to refrain,
a time to search and a time to give up,
a time to keep and a time to throw away,
a time to tear and a time to mend,
a time to be silent and a time to speak,
a time to love and a time to hate,
a time for war and a time for peace.

Genesis 6:3 tells us the number of years God intended for us to live on this earth: ***"My Spirit will not put up with humans for such a long time, for they are only mortal flesh. In the future, their normal lifespan will be no more than 120 years."*** I cannot recall too many times that I have heard of anyone living to be 120 years old. Maybe that is because we are not following the instructions given throughout the Word of God on how to live a long and healthy life.

By misunderstanding that disease processes such as diarrhea, fever, and inflammation are not only natural but necessary attempts by the body to regain optimum health, modern medicine frequently attempts to suppress these adaptive and eliminative processes with drugs and other invasive treatments. This may create deeper, more difficult problems by interfering with the body's self-healing mechanisms.

My goal is to help you become aware of how your body systems function; how to recognize and treat symptoms which are your body's attempt to correct imbalances and disharmony; and what you can do to restore and maintain your health naturally.

We are largely in control of how we feel and how we age; as well as how much pain or suffering we will endure in our later life. In other words, our lifestyle today will affect and determine our health, or lack thereof, in our retirement years.

Deuteronomy 5:33 tells us: *"Ye shall walk in all the ways which the LORD your God hath commanded you, that ye may live, and that it may be well with you, and that ye may prolong your days in the land which ye shall possess."* Micah 6:8 says: *"…And what doth the LORD require of thee, but to do justly, and to love mercy, and to walk humbly with thy God?"*

While doing research on how to cure my body of cancer naturally, I came across biblical principles in modern-day references—over and over. Such evidence encouraged me and helped strengthen my resolve. The Bible has the answers for staying healthy written down over 2,000 years ago!

Hebrews 13:8: *"Jesus Christ, the same yesterday, and today, and forever."* The Word of God is timeless. It speaks to every aspect of our lives.

The following sections will discuss modern-day scientific findings of treatments and cures that God provided when He made the world. Everything God created was GOOD. He filled the world with all we would ever need to live long and healthy lives. However, when sin came into the world, along with it came sickness, disease, and, inevitably, our physical death.

However, our loving Heavenly Father did not abandon us to this fate. John 3:16 tells us: *"For God so loved the world, that he gave his only begotten Son, that whosoever believeth in him should not perish, but have everlasting life."* Galatians 1:4 tells us, our Lord and Savior Jesus Christ *"Gave himself for our sins, that he might deliver us from this present evil world, according to the will of God and our Father."*

While Jesus walked the earth, He performed many healing miracles. He told us to do likewise in John 14:12-14: *"Verily, verily, I say unto you, He that believeth on me, the works that I do shall he do also; and greater works than these shall he do; because I go unto my Father. And whatsoever ye shall ask in my name, that will I do, that the Father may be glorified in the Son. If ye shall ask any thing in my name, I will do it."*

God says in Exodus 15:26 *If thou wilt diligently hearken to the voice of the LORD thy God, and wilt do that which is right in his sight, and wilt give ear to his commandments, and keep all his statutes,* (He says) ... *I am the LORD that <u>healeth</u> thee.*

If you are ill, first seek the Lord. The story of Asa warns about only seeking help from physicians.

2 Chronicles 16:12-13 (NIV) *In the thirty-ninth year of his reign Asa was afflicted with a disease in his feet. Though his disease was severe, even in his illness he did not seek help from the LORD, but only from the physicians. Then in the forty-first year of his reign Asa died and rested with his fathers.*

Put your faith in the healing power of God and do not rely solely on physicians. Even when the physicians give you no hope, recall Mark 5:25-29 *And a certain woman, which had an issue of blood twelve years, And had suffered many things of many physicians, and had spent all that she had, and was nothing bettered, but rather grew worse, When she had heard of Jesus, came in the press behind, and touched his garment. For she said, If I may touch but his clothes, I shall be whole. And straightway the fountain of her blood was dried up; and she felt in her body that she was healed of that plague."*

The woman's faith was rooted in her understanding of the Word of God from Malachi 4:2 *But unto you that fear my name shall the Sun of righteousness arise with healing in his wings. The word "wings"* has been interpreted as covering or garment. Her faith was such that if she only touched the hem of His garment she would be healed, just as the Scripture said.

Hebrews 11:6 tells us that we will be rewarded if we are faithful and diligently search the Scriptures for answers: *"But without faith it is impossible to please him: for he that cometh to God must believe that he is, and that he is a rewarder of them that diligently seek him."* Then John 1:14 tells us: *"Jesus was the word, And the Word was made flesh"* and *"He sent he word, and healed them"* Psalm 107:20.

Philippians 4:8

Finally, brethren, whatsoever things are true, whatsoever things are honest, whatsoever things are just, whatsoever things are pure, whatsoever things are lovely, whatsoever things are of good report; if there be any virtue, and if there be any praise, think on these things.

Acts 26:2

I think myself happy...

CHAPTER 13

MENTAL ATTITUDE

In Proverbs 18:14 (Amplified Bible), Solomon writes: *"The strong spirit of a man sustains him in bodily pain or trouble, but a weak and broken spirit who can raise up or bear?"*

And David says in Ecclesiastes 3:12-13: *"I know that there is nothing better for men than to be happy and do good while they live. That everyone may eat and drink, and find satisfaction in all his toil—this is the gift of God."*

Negative emotions and thoughts produce a destructive cycle of physical events that cause the breakdown of health and vitality which can eventually lead to the development of disease. It has been proven that emotions such as stress, anger, anxiety, or resentment cause the body to react in an unhealthy way. It can decrease the oxygen level in our cells and increase our body's acidity—thereby reducing our body's ability to fight disease. By releasing negative emotions, one can improve their health and even eliminate disease!

A positive mental attitude affects every aspect of our life: emotional, mental, and spiritual. If we are thinking positively, we are creating a life that is desirable. Psalm 55:22 tells us: ***"Cast thy burden upon the LORD, and he shall sustain thee: he shall never suffer the righteous to be moved."***

We can live happy lives and sustain our health by committing each day into God's hands, asking for His grace; thereby allowing the Holy Spirit to resolve our problems and guide us in the way the Lord would have us go. When we are truly centered in Christ, our inner conflicts can be eliminated, releasing positive energy that will improve our physical and mental health.

James Allen, author of As A Man Thinketh, realized this when he said: ***"The power of the human mind is so strong that it makes man possess an ability to mold his personality, create his future, build his destiny, and turn his dreams into reality."*** Likewise, the human mind, if focused on negative thoughts, including stress, anxiety, anger, and resentment, can lead to physical ailments. All of these have been shown to be a contributing factor in disorders and diseases such as cardiovascular disease, ulcers, blood pressure problems, headaches, respiratory problems,[1] and even cancer.

I believe if I had heeded this advice, I would not have developed breast cancer. As I mentioned earlier, I have always felt responsible for everyone else's happiness. I felt that I could solve every problem. Then came a time in my life when I couldn't seem to keep anyone happy, and the problems of my world were bigger than I was. If only I had let go of my problems, and let God take over!

God used breast cancer to teach me to trust in Him and to prepare me for the life He intended. Now, I can relate to 1 Peter 5:10 (Amplified Bible): *"And after you have suffered a little while, the God of all grace [Who imparts all blessing and favor], Who has called you to His [own] eternal glory in Christ Jesus, will Himself complete and make you what you ought to be, establish and ground you securely, and strengthen, and settle you."* Thank You, God!

---

1. Patel, Dimpel, *How Negative Thoughts Affect Your Life*, January 11, 2008

When we daily study the Word of God and speak to Him in prayer, it brings inner peace and insight into life's problems and decision-making. Our help is in Christ. Philippians 4:13 gives us personal security to trust the Lord for every aspect of our lives: ***"I can do all things through Christ who strengthens me."*** Do not become confused and frustrated with life. Let the Holy Spirit Who lives within each of God's children direct you through the problems of life. John 14:26-27 ***But the Comforter, which is the Holy Ghost, whom the Father will send in my name, he shall teach you all things, and bring all things to your remembrance, whatsoever I have said unto you. Peace I leave with you, my peace I give unto you: not as the world giveth, give I unto you. Let not your heart be troubled, neither let it be afraid.***

We do not have to worry about the failures of yesterday. Matthew 6:34 says: ***"Don't worry about tomorrow, tomorrow will take care of itself, and don't be concerned about yesterday, you can't recall it, it is past."*** The Apostle Paul instructs us in Philippians 3:13: ***"…Forgetting those things which are behind and reaching forward to those things which are ahead."*** Live for today! God will take care of your needs for tomorrow!

When God forgives, He also forgets. We must do likewise.

Luke 6:37 tells us: *"Judge not, and you shall not be judged. Condemn not, and you shall not be condemned. Forgive, and you will be forgiven."*

1 John 1:9 assures us: *"If we confess our sins, he is faithful and just to forgive us our sins, and to cleanse us from all unrighteousness."*

Life is filled with trials and temptations, sorrow and disappointments. However, the wisdom expressed in Proverbs 3:1-12 (The Message) reminds us: *"Don't lose your grip on Love and Loyalty. Tie them around your neck; carve their initials on your heart. Earn a reputation for living well in God's eyes and the eyes of the people. Trust God from the bottom of your heart; don't try to figure out everything on your own. Listen for God's voice in everything you do, everywhere you go; he's the one who will keep you on track. Don't assume that you know it all. Run to God! Run from evil! Your body will glow with health, your very bones will vibrate with life! Honor God with everything you own; give him the first and the best. Your barns will burst, your wine vats will brim over. But don't, dear friend, resent God's discipline; don't sulk under his loving correction. It's the child he loves that God corrects; a father's delight is behind all this."*

Ultimately, the best way to sustain your mental and

physical health is to be happy—don't stress, don't worry; forgive and forget when you have been wronged; and when you have done wrong, ask forgiveness. Pray without ceasing. Turn your cares over to the Lord. Do Not Worry! Remember, John 10:10 tells us: *"I am come that ye might have life and that ye might have it more abundantly."*

Remember also the wisdom from Matthew 6:25-34 *Therefore I tell you, do not worry about your life, what you will eat or drink; or about your body, what you will wear. Is not life more important than food, and the body more important than clothes? Look at the birds of the air; they do not sow or reap or store away in barns, and yet your heavenly Father feeds them. Are you not much more valuable than they? Who of you by worrying can add a single hour to his life? And why do you worry about clothes? See how the lilies of the field grow. They do not labor or spin. Yet I tell you that not even Solomon in all his splendor was dressed like one of these. If that is how God clothes the grass of the field, which is here today and tomorrow is thrown into the fire, will he not much more clothe you, O you of little faith? So do not worry, saying, 'What shall we eat?' or 'What shall we drink?' or 'What shall we wear?' For the pagans run after all these things, and your heavenly Father knows that you need them. But seek first his kingdom and his righteousness, and all these things will be given to you as well. Therefore do not worry about tomorrow, for tomorrow will worry about itself. Each day has enough trouble of its own.*

CHAPTER 14

DIET

"Those who fail to take the time to be healthy will ultimately have to take the time to be sick."
~ Dr. James Chappell

The Bible tells us that God created grass, herbs, and fruits on the third day of creation. He then specifically instructs us to consume them, because they were good. Genesis 1:12 *And the earth brought forth grass, and herb yielding seed after his kind, and the tree yielding fruit, whose seed was in itself, after his kind: and God saw that it was good.* Genesis 1:29 *And God said, Behold, I have given you every herb bearing seed, which is upon the face of all the earth, and every tree, in which is the fruit of a tree yielding seed; to you it shall be for meat.*

The ideal diet is one rich in vegetables, fruits, grains, legumes (beans), cold water ocean fish, olive oil, and, yes, a little red wine and red meat. The healthiest diet consists of seventy percent fresh raw fruits and vegetables, nuts and seeds. Raw food is much easer for your body to digest.

It passes through the digestive tract in one-half to one-third the time it takes for cooked food. Raw foods are also high in fiber and rich in enzymes, which are needed for the digestive system to work efficiently. Enzymes are necessary to break down food particles so they can be utilized for energy. A lack of digestive enzymes can be a factor in food allergies, bloating, belching, gas, bowel disorders, abdominal cramping, and heartburn.

Only about thirty percent of one's diet should be made up of cooked foods, grains, legumes, and meats. Nearly every food preparation process reduces the amount of nutrients in food. When raw foods are exposed to temperatures above 118 degrees, they start to rapidly break down. Many nutrients are lost in the cooking process; and once enzymes are exposed to heat, they are no longer able to provide the function for which they were designed.

Another important reason to include fruits and vegetables in one's diet is the body's need for fiber. According to The Institute of Medicine, children and adults should consume 14 grams of fiber for every 1,000 calories of food they eat each day. A fiber deficiency increases your risk of high cholesterol, cardiovascular disease, high blood sugar (which can lead to diabetes), obesity, colon cancer, hemorrhoids, and constipation. Irregular bowel movements do not properly flush waste from our body and allow toxins to build up in our system.

This toxic overload can be the cause of migraine headaches and, now I have found, even breast cancer. Physicians Nicholas L. Petrakis and Eileen B. King of the University of California, writing in Lancet, have found that women who have two or fewer bowel movements per week have four times the risk of breast disease (benign or malignant) as women who have one or more bowel movements per day.

Consuming nutrition-rich foods ensures that the vitamins and minerals they contain will be processed completely. When too large a quantity of food is consumed at one time, or when high-dosage supplements are consumed, the body cannot process the nutrition fast enough—causing the precious vitamins and minerals to be lost because the body cannot absorb such large quantities. Also, if there is inadequate water available to cleanse one's body tissues, a toxic buildup may result. This danger does not exist when we introduce nutrients into the body through natural raw foods. The nutrition one consumes from food is more easily absorbed by the body.

The Word of God expressly warns against abstaining from meat because of fear or false doctrine.

1 Timothy 4:1-5 assures us of the goodness of all that

God has created: *"But the Spirit saith expressly, that in later times some shall fall away from the faith, giving heed to seducing spirits and doctrines of demons, through the hypocrisy of men that speak lies, branded in their own conscience as with a hot iron; forbidding to marry, and commanding to abstain from meats, which God created to be received with thanksgiving by them that believe and know the truth. For every creature of God is good, and nothing is to be rejected, if it be received with thanksgiving: for it is sanctified through the word of God and prayer."*

Paul also instructs in 1 Corinthians 10:24-26 *Nobody should seek his own good, but the good of others. Eat anything sold in the meat market without raising questions of conscience for "The earth is the Lord's, and everything in it."* And Luke instructs in Acts 27:34 *Wherefore, I pray you to take some meat: for this is for your health...*

I know from my own experience that when I gave up red meat, as recommended by the Naturopath for the treatment of cancer, my energy level plummeted. I was introduced to Dr. Peter D'Adamo's book, Eat Right 4 Your Type, and realized I was not meant to be a vegetarian. Dr. D'Adamo had interviewed 6,617 individuals who reported their results from following the Blood Type Diet for a period of just one month. The report found that three out of four people had significant improvement in a variety of health conditions including weight loss, improvements in digestive function, resistance to stress, overall energy, and mental clarity. I have "O" blood type and found that I was one of those that saw a drastic improvement in my energy level and over all mood.

The survey also showed the same percentages of positive results across all blood types. Type "O" individuals, who follow a higher protein (meat), lower carbohydrate diet were as likely to report positive results as Type "A" individuals, who follow a lower fat, plant-based diet, or types "B" and "AB" individuals, who follow a more omnivorous (both plant and animal- based foods) diet.

The Apostle Mark again tells us that all food is good, Mark 7:18-23 *So He said to them, "Are you thus without understanding also? Do you not perceive that whatever enters a man from outside cannot defile him, because it does not enter his heart but his stomach, and is eliminated, thus purifying all foods. And He said, "What comes out of a man; that defiles a man. For from within, out of the heart of men, proceed evil thoughts, adulteries, fornications, murders, thefts, covetousness, wickedness, deceit, lewdness, an evil eye, blasphemy, pride, foolishness. All these evil things come from within and defile a man.*

Our concern should be about what is in our heart and mind. What we think and speak is far more destructive to our health than the food we eat or what we drink. James Allen, author of *As A Man Thinketh*, knew this when he wrote: "As a man thinketh in his heart so is he." A sick mind, a broken heart, harbored feelings of anger or resentment, will lead to a diseased physical state.

1 Corinthians 13 tells us that Love is the most important thing it is universally the greatest gift. *"Love is patient, love is kind, it isn't jealous, it doesn't brag, it isn't arrogant, it isn't rude, it doesn't seek its own advantage, it isn't irritable, it doesn't keep a record of complaints, it isn't happy with injustice, but it is happy with the truth. Love puts up with all things, trusts in all things, hopes for all things, endures all things... Love never fails. Now faith, hope, and love remain—these three things—and the greatest of these is love."*

CHAPTER 15

WHEN IS ABSTINENCE REQUIRED?

1 Thessalonians 5:22
"Abstain from all appearance of evil."

There are certainly instances when it is appropriate to refrain from certain foods or beverages—whether it is a vow of abstinence or during a time of fasting, cleansing, or as part of a healing diet. Whatever the reason, our commitment needs to be taken as seriously as a vow and always and only to honor God. Romans 14:6 ... **He that eateth, eateth to the Lord, for he giveth God thanks; and he that eateth not, to the Lord he eateth not, and giveth God thanks.**

When someone pledges, or resolves solemnly to strictly observe certain dietary guidelines in order to give their body the necessary nutrition to heal naturally. It is crucial that they do not grow weary, but continue to purse God's guidance and adhere to the vow they have made; believing that God will honor their commitment just as He did those in Bible days. The Bible tells us, in Ecclesiastes 5:5 (NIV) ***It is better not to vow than to make a vow and not fulfill it.***

According to Dr. Budwig, "It is possible to restore health in a few months at most, 90% of the time". However, her research has shown "that those who break the dietary rules, eating preserved meats, candy, etc, will sometimes grow rapidly worse and cannot be saved after they come back from their spree."

In James 2:20 we read: *"Faith without works is dead."* This statement confirms that faith is valueless if we do not act on our beliefs. Our Heavenly Father can and does perform miracles of healing. However; we must be willing and committed to do our part. By making healthy changes to our diet and life style we are in essence acting on our faith. There are numerous accounts in the Bible of extraordinary men and women that were instructed by God to abnegate certain foods and beverages and make other physical sacrifices for a period of time, when they would be separate unto the Lord. Specific instructions to those commissioned to the highest calling of Nazarite priests are listed in Numbers 6.

Those who vowed to God and adhered strictly to that

vow were given great physical and spiritual strength. Judges 13-16 tells the story of the life of Samson. His life also illustrates the blessings are removed if the vow is not honored.

John the Baptist was also designated as a Nazarite priest. His amazing story is told in Luke 1, **His Father, Zacharias was told by an Angel of the Lord: "For he shall be great in the sight of the Lord, and shall drink neither wine nor strong drink; and he shall be filled with the Holy Ghost, even from his mother's womb."**

Then, the first chapter of Daniel, tells of the vow Daniel, Hananiah, Mishael, and Azariah made when captured by Nebuchadnezzar, king of Babylon. Daniel 1: 8 **But Daniel purposed in his heart that he would not defile himself with the portion of the king's meat, nor with the wine which he drank: let them give us pulse (raw leguminous plants, peas, beans, etc.1) to eat, and water to drink... God blessed them with great wisdom and honored their vow; And in all matters of wisdom and understanding, that the king enquired of them, he found them ten times better than all the magicians and astrologers that were in all his realm.**

The Word of God instructs us to seek the Lord's favor and not the favor of men in Colossians 3 **And whatsoever**

ye do, do it heartily, as to the Lord, and not unto men; Knowing that of the Lord ye shall receive the reward of the inheritance: for ye serve the Lord Christ.

Often, others do not understand one's vows made to honor God, nor do they appreciate the limitations one imposes on oneself as part of a dietary commitment. 1 Corinthians 2:14 says: ***"But the natural man receiveth not the things of the Spirit of God: for they are foolishness unto him: neither can he know them, because they are spiritually discerned."***

Examples of man's lack of understanding are given in the way John the Baptist and Jesus were perceived. Luke 7:33 tells us that ***"John the Baptist came neither eating bread nor drinking wine; and ye (they) say, He hath a devil."***

When Jesus came eating and drank, they called him a winebibber. When Jesus came, freeing men of dietary restrictions, he was rejected and mocked by the Pharisees and lawyers that did not believe. Luke 7:34 ***The Son of Man is come eating and drinking; and ye say, Behold a gluttonous man, and a winebibber, a friend of publicans and sinners!***

If we as Christians seek to model our lives after Christ, we too will be misunderstood, mocked and ridiculed. Jesus tells us in Matthew 10:24-26 (Common English Bible) that we can expect to be call even worse than He was. *"Disciples aren't greater than their teacher, and slaves aren't greater than their master. It's enough for disciples to be like their teacher and slaves like their master. If they have called the head of the house Beelzebul, it's certain that they will call the members of his household by even worse names. Therefore, don't be afraid of those people because nothing is hidden that won't be revealed, and nothing secret that won't be brought out into the open."*

Psalms 104:14-15

*"He causeth the grass to grow for the cattle,
and herb for the service of man: that he may bring
forth food out of the earth;
And wine that maketh glad the heart of man,
and oil to make his face to shine,
and bread which strengtheneth man's heart."*

CHAPTER 16

WINE AND SPIRITS

The Apostle Paul instructed in 1 Timothy 5:23 ***Drink no longer water, but use a little wine for thy stomach's sake and thine often infirmities.***

Research has now proven that drinking a modest amount of wine or other alcoholic beverages is actually good for your health. It can lower your bad cholesterol, increase your good cholesterol, lower your blood pressure, increase your bone density, reduce your chance of kidney stones, increase your memory, and extend your life expectancy.

Wine, particularly those made with red grapes, contains a substance called Resveratrol. This naturally-occurring phenol, which also inhibits cancer growth, has a proven ability to protect against atherosclerosis and coronary heart disease.

The Mayo Clinic published information stating "the alcohol and certain substances in red wine called antioxidants may help prevent heart disease by increasing levels of "good" cholesterol and protect against artery damage."

The medical journal, Cell Metabolism, suggested Resveratrol helps keep the bones, eyes, kidneys, heart, and other muscles healthier as one ages. The recommended consumption: one [1] or two [2] glasses of beer or wine or one and one half [1½] ounces of liquor—per day.

New Science Magazine cites a University College of London study whereby data was collected from more than 12,000 mothers and children in the United Kingdom over a period of seven years. Apparently: "kids whose mothers had one to two alcoholic drinks per week during pregnancy had fewer cognitive and behavioral problems by age three than those of woman who abstained."

John 2:1-11 gives the account of Jesus' first miracle—turning water to wine. There is a second account in John 4:46 **So Jesus came again into Cana of Galilee, where he made the water wine.** Jesus did not condemn drinking, He, himself drank wine, and He would never have miraculously produced more wine at the wedding ceremony when they ran out, if it was bad. Remember, all things God created are good.

The ceremony of Holy Communion is given to us by Christ Himself, so that we might remember and participate in His last supper with His disciples, before his arrest and crucifixion. He commands us to observe it. Do this "in remembrance of me." Luke 22:19. Paul writes in 1 Cor. 11:24 *And when he (Jesus) had given thanks, he brake it (the bread), and said, Take, eat: this is my body, which is broken for you: this do in remembrance of me. 25 After the same manner also he took the cup (wine), when he had supped, saying, this cup is the new testament in my blood: this do ye, as oft as ye drink it, in remembrance of me. 26 For as often as ye eat this bread, and drink this cup, ye do shew the Lord's death till he come.*

Every time we partake in Holy Communion, we recall the sacrifice Jesus made for us on the cross and the promises he made.

Isaiah 53:5 *But he was wounded for our transgressions; he was bruised for our iniquities: the chastisement of our peace was upon him; and with his stripes we are healed.*

1 Peter 2:24 *Who his own self bare our sins in his own body on the tree, that we, being dead to sins, should live unto righteousness: by whose stripes ye were healed.*

CHAPTER 17

THE DANGER OF FOOD ADDITIVES

Jesus freed us from dietary restrictions imposed in Old Testament law, and the Word tells us that all fruits, vegetables, grains, seeds, and meats have been made by God to be eaten and enjoyed by mankind.

Unfortunately, today many of the foods and beverages we consume are laced with additives, preservatives, and food coloring. The processing methods add hydrogenated oils, stabilizers, and flavor enhancers that are manmade and unhealthy for human consumption. In order to increase production, herbicides, pesticides, and chemical fertilizers are added to soil and sprayed on the fields.

Toxic build-up from consuming large quantities of preservatives, food additives and pesticides, have been linked to developmental disorders and other serious diseases.

These include but are not limited to:

Cancer	Cardio-vascular disease
Impaired Immune system	Hormonal Imbalances
ADHD	Hyperactivity
Learning Disorders	Autism
Brain Fog	Obesity
Headaches	Joint Pain and Stiffness
Migraines	Anemia
Nasal Congestion and Mucus	Skin Rashes
Dark Circles under the Eyes	Brown Blotches on the Skin
Muscular Sclerosis	Rheumatoid Arthritis

Our body stores chemicals and toxins in our fat. Thereby, explaining the huge increase in obesity amongst those that consume the greatest quantities of processed foods and the largest number of meals eaten at fast food restaurants. It has been proven that environmental toxins in fat cause obesity, diabetes and cancer.

Weight gain is more than a calories problem.
It is a toxin problem.

According to J. K.Paulsen, M.D. a Bariatric Physician "The body naturally manufactures fat in abundance to incarcerate and absorb chemicals and toxins that accumulate over time. As you cleanse the body, one can expect fat and inches to be substantially reduced."

"The Environmental Protection Agency has monitored human exposure to toxic environmental chemicals since 1972 when they began the National Human Adipose Tissue Survey. They found that five of what are known to be the most toxic chemicals were found in 100% of all samples.

"Nine more chemicals were found in 91-98% of samples: "Polychlorinated biphenyls (PCBs) were found in 83% of the population".[1]

I strongly recommend that everyone eat raw, organic foods and meat from wild game or grass fed livestock whenever possible and avoid processed foods, because, they can cause serious side-effects and toxicity. Foods consumed in their natural state give you the full benefit of God's design to keep your body in good health.

The chart below has been compiled of information I discovered while doing research for a natural cancer cure. It lists some of the most common food additives and their known side effects.

1. *Source: Mark Hyman, Systems Biology,Toxins,Obesity,and Functional Medicine. 13th International Symposium of The Institute for Functional Medicine*

I became extremely careful when grocery shopping, reading labels and asking questions at the meat department and even at the farmers market. Avoiding harmful food additives was an important step in my recovery from cancer.

Chemical's Names:	Chemical's Typically found in	Potential Health Effects
Hormones	Meat Products (fresh and processed) Cow's milk and cow's milk products (cheese, yogurt, etc)	Linked to an increased risk of breast, colon, prostate and lung cancer. 29 Has also been linked to larger than normal breasts and young girls starting periods earlier than normal. 30
Antibiotics	Fresh and Processed Meat Products	Linked to antibiotic resistance in humans. High levels of nitrofuran, an antibiotic known to cause cancer. 31
Chlorine	Public water systems and swimming pools	Chlorinated water linked to the aggravation and cause of respiratory diseases like asthma. The most serious side effect is Alzheimer's disease.
Fluoride	Public water systems, toothpaste, mouth washes	Fluoride Linked to cancer, diabetes, thyroid and neurological disorders, hormonal imbalances, heart disease, arthritis and osteoporosis

29 Jeffery M. Smith, *Genetic Roulette: The Documented Health Risks of Genetically Engineered Foods* (Fairfield, IA: Yes Books, 2007) 157.
30 Cohen, Robert, *Early Sexual Maturity and Milk Hormones*, health101.org,
31 Martin Khor, *The dangers of antibiotics in animal feed*, Third World Network 124

Aluminum	Public water systems, toothpaste, mouth washes	Aluminum has been linked to Parkinson-type diseases. A neuron-toxic hazard and
Glutamino Acid (MSG) Monsodium Glutamite	Found in many processed foods often will be listed as (spice) in the ingredient list.	Behavioral problems in children, attention deficit hyperactivity disorder or emotional problems. Children often undergo a remarkable change when MSG is eliminated from their diet
Benzene (preservative)	Can be found in beverages that contain both ascorbic acid (vitamin C) and sodium benzoate	Known carcinogen. Benzene causes harmful effects on the bone marrow and can causea decrease in red blood cells leading to anemia. It can also cause excessive bleedingand an affect the immune system. 32
Artificial Sweeteners	Packaged and processed foods, diet foods, and sugar free foods	Linked to cancers, hyperactivity / ADHD / learning disability affect
Methylene chloride - a solvent used to remove caffeine from coffee.	Decaffeinated Coffee	Proven carcinogenic that is toxic to lungs, the nervous system, liver, mucous membranes, central nervous system (CNS). Repeated or prolonged exposure to the substance can produce target organs damage. 33

32 Avianweb.com/diseasescausedbytoxin.html
33 Avianweb.com/diseasescausedbytoxin.html

Tartrazine aka FD&C Yellow No:5; CI Acid Yellow 23, CI Food Yellow 4. Coal tar dye.	Sodas, sweets, jams, cereals, snack foods, canned fish, packaged soups	Cancer probability. Known to provoke asthma attacks and urticaria (nettle rash) in children. May cause altered states of perception and behavior, uncontrolled hyper agitation and confusion; wakefulness in young children. Is also known to inhibit zinc metabolism and interfere with digestive enzymes.
Yellow 2G, Acid yellow 17, CI Food yellow 5, Coal tar dye, artificial color	Soft drinks	May cause asthma, rashes and hyperactivity
Sunset Yellow FCF, Orange Yellow S, FD&C Yellow No: 6, CI Food yellow 3 artificial color	Cereals, bakery, sweets, snack foods, ice cream/ candy, drinks and canned fish, orange squash, jelly, jam, cakes, soups, desert mixes, yogurt, sauces	Can provoke allergic reactions such as abdominal pain, hyperactivity, hives and nasal congestion. Potentially dangerous to asthmatics. Bronchoconstriction, kidney tumours, and chromosomal damage. It also produces urticaria, swelling of the blood vessels and gastric upset.
FD&C Red No: 40 artificial orange-red color	Sweets, cakes, biscuits, drinks, condiments, medications	Has been connected with cancer.

Indigotine, Indigo carmine, FD&C Blue No:2, synthetic coal tar dye, artificial color	Milk deserts, sweets, biscuits, ice creams, baked goods, confectionary	May cause nausea, vomiting, high blood pressure, skin rashes, breathing problems, brain tumors and other allergic reactions **34**
Brilliant blue FCF, FD&C Blue Dye No: 1, CI Acid blue 9, CI Food blue 2, CI Pigment blue24artificial color	Dairy products, sweets and drinks	Can cause hyperactivity, skin rashes, chromosomal damage and broncho-constriction
Sulphur dioxide (SO2)- a preservative used in gaseous form or as salts (sulfites)	Sulphured dried fruit, fruit drinks, wine, meat, and as a processing aid to control physical properties of flour	Protects vitamin C, but destroys vitamin B1. May cause asthma and anaphylactic shock. Dangerous for asthma, allergy sufferers. Has resulted in deaths. Banned on fresh fruits and vegetables.

34 Avianweb.com/diseasescausedbytoxin.html#benzene.

CHAPTER 18

WATER

The Bible speaks of water hundreds of times. The Word of God is referred to as *Living Water.* In John 7:38, Jesus said: **"He who believes in Me, as the Scripture has said, out of his heart will flow rivers of living water."**

It is through the baptism with water that grace is conferred on a believer. No matter what is in a person's past, baptism starts anew the covenantal relationship between God and the person being baptized. Matthew 3:11 **I indeed baptize you with water unto repentance, but He who is coming after me is mightier than I, whose sandals I am not worthy to carry. He will baptize you with the Holy Spirit and fire.**

Water was also used repeatedly in miraculous healings. John 9:11 **He answered and said, A man that is called**

Jesus made clay, and anointed mine eyes, and said unto me, Go to the pool of Siloam, and wash: and I went and washed, and I received sight." John 5:2-4 *Now there is at Jerusalem by the sheep market a pool, which is called in the Hebrew tongue Bethesda,* (there) *lay a great multitude of impotent folk, of blind, halt, withered, waiting for the moving of the water. For an angel went down at a certain season into the pool, and troubled the water: whosoever then first after the troubling of the water stepped in was made whole of whatsoever disease he had.*

Water has long been known to promote health due to its restorative and detoxifying properties. Without water, life is impossible. Every living thing depends on water to survive. The human body is estimated to be about sixty to seventy percent water—blood is eighty-three percent water; our brain is seventy-seven to seventy-eight percent water. We human beings can only survive without water for approximately three days as our body needs to constantly replace the water lost due to perspiration and normal bodily functions. In order to remain healthy, one's daily diet needs to include a minimum of one ounce of water for every two pounds of body weight. Approximately eight [8], eight-ounce glasses of water are required for an individual weighing 128 pounds. Without adequate water intake, the body cannot regulate its temperature or provide the means for nutrients to travel to all its organs. Water also transports oxygen to our cells, removes waste, and protects our joints and organs.

Fortunately, the foods we consume contribute to our water intake. Leafy vegetables, root vegetables, and sprouts generally consist of ninety [90] to ninety-five [95] percent water, and fruits eighty [80] to ninety [90] percent water. Therefore, by eating one cup of vegetables or fruit, you will consume almost one cup of water.[1]

Dairy products are also a great source of water. Milk is eighty-eight [88] percent water; yogurt eighty [80] percent water. By consuming eight [8] to sixteen [16] ounces per day, one is able to easily increase their fluid intake. Then by replacing cow's milk with fresh goat's milk, one receiving a complete protein source which contains all the essential amino acids as well as a great source of calcium and vitamin C.

Goat's milk is one of the best known foods for regenerating the cells of the body. It is also well know as a healing remedy for stomach, colon, intestinal and arthritic like conditions.

1. Brooke, Dorothea, *Meeting Hydration without actually drinking water*, Associated content, Institute of Medicine of the National Academies, August 28, 2007

It is one of the best foods for rebuilding the nervous system, brain, and improving mental function. Another added benefit of goat's milk is that it is much lower in fat content than cow's milk. Its fat globules are one ninth the size of cow's milk, which makes it easier to digest and it is naturally homogenized.

Dry ingredients, such as beans, grains, rice and pasta, also become water-rich foods when cooked. This is because they act as sponges absorbing the water in which they are prepared. A cup of these products also contains nearly two-thirds cup of water. Even lean meats, especially poultry and fish, are generally 62 to 70 percent water.

Caffeine and caffeinated beverages such as coffee, tea, soft drinks and energy drink, act as diuretics, which increases the excretion of water from ones body. Therefore, caffeinated beverages cannot be included when considering your water intake because you will actually lose through urination, more water than you consume due to the diuretic effect of caffeine.

Common side-effects of over-consumption of diuretics or caffeinated beverages are the loss of potassium and magnesium. Listed below are some of the serious side-effects of low potassium levels, including but not limited to:

- fatigue
- muscle weakness and cramps
- intestinal paralysis, which may lead to bloating
- constipation

The best foods to replenish your body's potassium levels include:

- cold water ocean fish
- oranges
- tomatoes
- avocados
- dates
- carrots
- prunes
- apricots
- bananas
- figs

Low magnesium levels can cause some or all of the following:

- sensitivity to noise
- irritability
- confusion
- trembling
- insomnia
- nervousness
- mental depression
- twitching
- apprehension
- muscle weakness and cramps in the toes, feet, legs, or fingers

The best foods to restore your body's magnesium levels include:
- whole-grain breads and cereals
- beans
- nuts
- cocoa
- corn
- bananas
- dark green vegetables

It has been documented that many serious health conditions are linked to dehydration. Some of the most common are listed below. If you suffer from any of the following conditions, you may very well be dehydrated and, therefore, could cure your condition with simply drinking enough water and increasing your intake of high moisture, nutritious foods.

Conditions linked to dehydration:
- dermatitis
- diabetes
- high blood pressure
- obesity
- tension headaches
- restless leg syndrome
- constipation
- dry skin and hair
- indigestion
- osteoporosis
- muscle cramps
- fatigue

There is growing scientific evidence linking increased water intake with a reduced risk of major illness.

Consuming adequate amounts of water significantly reduces the risk of developing kidney stones and is even instrumental in the prevention of cancer and heart disease. The easiest way to monitor whether you are getting enough water is to keep an eye on the color of your urine. Very pale yellow urine ensures you are well-hydrated. If your urine color strays into darker tones, particularly if it starts to smell a bit, it's time to reach for the water.

1 Timothy 4:8

*For bodily exercise profits a little,
but godliness is profitable for all things,
having promise of the life that now is
and of that which is to come.*

CHAPTER 19

EXERCISE

Jesus instructs us in Jeremiah 9:24 ***Exercise loving kindness, judgment, and righteousness, in the earth: for in these things I delight, saith the LORD.*** Then in 1 Timothy 4 the Bible specifically speaks of physical exercise ***"7 But refuse profane and old wives' fables, and exercise thyself rather unto godliness. 8 For bodily exercise is profitable for a little; but godliness is profitable for all things, having promise of the life which now is, and of that which is to come."*** The Word of God instructs that our faith and trust should be in the Lord—not in the food we eat or on a strict regimen of exercise.

Throughout the Bible, the words *"work"* and *"walk"* are used hundreds of times. God intends for us to be active in our faith and in our physical lives.

James 2:20 tells us, *"That faith without works is dead."* And in Isaiah 57:2 *Those who walk uprightly enter into peace.*

Research has shown that people who live active lives especially those who walk regularly have fewer incidences of cancer, heart disease, stroke, diabetes, and many other debilitating diseases. They live longer and have continued mental health and experience great spiritual benefit.

The benefits of exercise are obvious; especially important in this day and age with so many sedentary jobs offering limited activity. Much of today's leisure time is also sedentary—dominated by the use of computers, telephones, and televisions. Lack of physical activity has contributed to a generation of obesity and disease.

Listed below is a sampling of some of the health conditions that will be improved, many even cured, by a simple exercise regimen:

- Improved digestion.
- Enhanced quality of sleep—a good night's sleep can improve your concentration, productivity, and mood.
- A brisk thirty-minute walk helps us calm down after a stressful event.
- Increased muscle strength and energy.
- Enables weight loss and keeps it off by burning extra calories.

- Help prevent Type 2 diabetes by improving your body's ability to use insulin. Normally, insulin is released from the pancreas when the amount of sugar (glucose) in the blood increases, such as after eating. Insulin stimulates the liver and muscles to take in excess glucose. This results in a lowering of the blood sugar level.
- When exercising, the body needs extra energy or fuel (in the form of glucose) for the exercising muscles. With continued moderate exercise, your muscles take up glucose at almost twenty times the normal rate. This lowers blood sugar levels.
- Improves mental focus and concentration.
- Reduces your risk of diseases such as Alzheimer's and senility.
- Regular exercise, especially weight-bearing exercise, reduces the risk of osteoporosis, and can even reverse it by building bone tissue
- Reduce the risk of Breast Cancer by up to 60%. Estradiol and pro- gesterone, two ovarian hormones which are linked to breast cancer tumor production, are lowered in the body by exercise. Fat has long been known to be a catalyst in the production of estrogen (estradiol). Regular exercise burns body fat thus decreasing the rate of estrogen production and the risk of breast cancer.

- Makes you more limber and improves endurance.
- Endorphins ("feel good" hormones) are increased through exercise. Nothing improves mood and suppresses depression better than endorphins.
- Improves circulation and helps reduce blood pressure.
- Alleviates menstrual cramps.
- Enhances coordination and balance.
- Improves posture.
- Helps manage high blood pressure and improves cholesterol levels.
- Regular physical activity boosts high-density lipoprotein (HDL) [the "good" cholesterol] while decreasing triglycerides.
- Eases, and even eliminates, some back problems and pain.
- Keeps your blood flowing smoothly by lowering the buildup of plaque in your arteries.
- Reduces joint discomfort and makes the body more agile.
- Increases your range of motion.
- Enhances the immune system thereby reducing your risk of infection and the likelihood of contracting a cold or flu.

- Improves liver function which aids in detoxification.
- Physical activity delivers oxygen and nutrients to your tissues. In fact, regular physical activity helps your entire cardiovascular system — the circulation of blood through your heart and blood vessels makes them work more efficiently. When your heart and lungs work more efficiently, you'll have more energy.
- Helps to alleviate varicose veins.

Everyone would benefit from finding a physical activity they enjoy and engaging in it for at least twenty minutes three times per week.

CHAPTER 20

SUNLIGHT

In the first chapter of Genesis, the fourth day of the creation: *"God made two great lights; the greater light to rule the day, and the lesser light to rule the night: he made the stars also. And God set them in the firmament of the heaven to give light upon the earth, And to rule over the day and over the night, and to divide the light from the darkness: and God saw that it was good."*

God made the sun, and everything that He made is good and to be enjoyed by His people. Ecclesiastes 5:18 tells us: *"Behold that which I have seen: it is good and comely for one to eat and to drink, and to enjoy the good of all his labour that he taketh under the sun all the days of his life, which God giveth him: for it is his portion."*

The human body was designed by God to synthesize vitamin D in the skin when exposed to ultraviolet B (UVB) radiation from the sun. Sunlight exposure provides people with their entire vitamin D requirement. Unfortunately, there is a growing impact on the production of vitamin D in the body, because of the use of sunscreen. According to the *Linus Pauling Institute*, "the application of sunscreen with an SPF factor of 8 reduces production of vitamin D by 95%." Vitamin D helps maintain bone density, healthy bone growth, and helps maintain the normal functioning of the nervous system. It is crucially important in aiding the body's absorption of calcium. Without sufficient vitamin D, calcium supplements are almost useless. Vitamin D insufficiency is a contributing factor in osteoporosis, as calcium absorption cannot be maximized. Vitamin D's purpose is to maintain blood levels of calcium in the correct, normal range and to tell the body to absorb more calcium from food as needed. Osteoporosis is strongly associated with low Vitamin D levels.

Doctors know low levels of vitamin D are linked to certain kinds of cancers, as well as to diabetes and asthma, now, new research also shows that vitamin D can kill human cancer cells.

JoEllen Welsh, a researcher with the State University of New York at Albany, has studied the effects of vitamin D for twenty-five years. She found when human breast cancer cells were treated with vitamin D; within a few days, half the cancer cells shriveled up and died. *"What happens is that vitamin D enters the cells and triggers the cell death process,"* she told **Good Morning America**. *"It's similar to what we see when we treat cells with Tamoxifen,* [a drug used to treat breast cancer][1] *but without the side effects."*

In Traditional Chinese Medicine (TCM) cancer is often viewed as a symptom of a circulation problem. This hypothesis is strengthened by the fact that many factors that decrease the risk of cancer also thin the blood. These include sunshine, exercise, aspirin, heparin (a prescription anticoagulant), antibiotics, olive oil, fish oil, turmeric, vitamin E and garlic.[2]

Research also shows that Vitamin D is *extremely* important in regulating the immune system and controlling the expression of thousands of genes.

Vitamin D deficiency could be a major contributing factor to the current epidemic of cancer and diabetes. It has also been found that a higher intake of vitamin D can help lower the risk of certain cancers such as breast, prostate, and colorectal.

1. Clarke, Suzan, ABC News, *In Tests, Vitamin D Shrinks Breast Cancer Cells*, February 22, 2010
2. http://www.ctds.info/natthinners.html

The lack of Vitamin D contributes to chronic fatigue and depression, and to Seasonal Affective Disorder (SAD). It also is the cause of some cases of congenital heart failure. The article *'Mothers to be, better get your Vitamin D'* outlines the case that prenatal vitamin D deficiency may be linked to problems later in life such as:

Schizophrenia

Osteoporosis

Decayed Teeth

The chart below lists some of the best food sources of Vitamin D:

Goat's Milk	**Fortified Milk Products**
Cod Liver Oil	Butter
Lard	Lamb Liver
Atlantic Herring	Beef Tallow
Eastern Oysters	Pork Liver
Catfish	Beef Liver
Skinless Sardines	Beef Tripe
Canned Mackerel	Beef Kidney
Smoked Chinook Salmon	Chicken Livers
Sturgeon	Small Clams
Shrimp	Blue Crab
Egg Yolk	Crayfish/Crawdads
(One yolk contains 24 IU)	Northern Lobster

Minimal sun exposure of at least 10 - 15 minutes, 3 times a week during the spring, summer, and fall, in the middle of the day from 11 a.m. to 2 p.m., on the face and arms, will provide enough vitamin D for the average individual. This sun exposure will also allow for storage of excess vitamin D during the winter when UVB rays will not reach some areas.[3]

For people who live in latitudes around 40 degrees north or 40 degrees south of the equator, there is insufficient UVB radiation available for the skin to synthesize enough into vitamin D during the winter months.[4]

Vitamin D is fat soluble, which means it can be stored in your body for times when sun exposure is not available. It is possible when taking supplements to overdose on Vitamin D which causes toxicity. However, an overdose on Vitamin D *NEVER* occurs with naturally occurring vitamin D in foods or from sunlight.

---

3. Boston University, Dr. Michael Holick
4. Linus Apuling, Oregon State university

Ecclesiastes 11:7

"Truly the light is sweet, and a pleasant thing it is for the eyes to behold the sun."

Psalm 37:7

"Rest in the LORD, and wait patiently for him."

CHAPTER 21

REST

Sleep is essential to good health, because it refreshes the body and the mind. If you get enough sleep regularly every night, you will feel restored, refreshed, and able to work better. During our waking hours, our nerve cells are constantly active and become fatigued. Sleep gives the cells of our body an opportunity to repair themselves. In the first book of the Bible, Genesis 2 tells us that even God rested after creating the earth: ***"Thus the heavens and the earth were finished, and all the host of them. And on the seventh day God ended his work which he had made; and he rested on the seventh day from all his work which he had made. And God blessed the seventh day, and sanctified it: because that in it he had rested from all his work which God created and made."***

Then, God instructs us also to rest on the Sabbath and to allow our servants, the alien in the land, and even our cattle to rest.

Exodus 35:2: *"For six days, work is to be done, but the seventh day shall be your holy day, a Sabbath of rest to the LORD."*

Leviticus 23:3 *There are six days when you may work, but the seventh day is a Sabbath of rest, a day of sacred assembly. You are not to do any work; wherever you live, it is a Sabbath to the LORD.*

Deuteronomy 5:14 *But the seventh day is a Sabbath to the LORD your God. On it you shall not do any work, neither you, nor your son or daughter, nor your manservant or maidservant, nor your ox, your donkey or any of your animals, nor the alien within your gates, so that your manservant and maidservant may rest, as you do.*

Exodus 34:21 *Six days you shall labor, but on the seventh day you shall rest; even during the plowing season and harvest you must rest.*

Without adequate rest, a person may experience significant reductions in performance and alertness by as much as thirty-two percent. Your cognitive ability— to think and process information—is also reduced. Inadequate rest is also associated with numerous serious medical illnesses including but not limited to:

High blood pressure

Cardiovascular disease

Stroke

Obesity

Diabetes

Psychiatric problems, including depression and other mood disorders

Attention Deficit Disorder (ADD)

Mental impairment

Fetal and childhood growth retardation[1]

We were created with the ability to heal and recover from disease while we rest. It is during deep sleep that the production of growth hormone is at its peak. Growth hormone speeds the absorption of nutrients and amino acids into our cells and aids the healing of tissues throughout our body. This hormone also stimulates our bone marrow, where our immune system cells are born. Researchers at the *National Cancer Institute* have reported that women who consistently sleep less than seven hours a night have a 47% higher risk of developing cancer.

[1] 28 Breus, Michael J., PhD, MD, *Chronic Sleep Deprivation May Harm Health*, WebMD

Melatonin, often called the sleep hormone, is also produced during sleep. This hormone inhibits tumors from growing, prevents viral infections, stimulates one's immune system, increases antibodies in our saliva, has antioxidant properties, and enhances the quality of sleep.[2]

According to the *National Sleep Foundation*, the average adult requires seven to nine hours of sleep each night; children require even more. The most effective hours to sleep are between 10 p.m. and 6 a.m. In order to receive the full benefit of proper rest, the room should be well-ventilated, completely dark, and quiet.

Adequate rest is so important to our overall health that it is *ordered* by God. The Bible assures us repeatedly that God is with us *as* we rest. In fact, peaceful rest is a gift *from* Him.

---

2. William Collinge, M.P.H., Ph.D., *Sleep's healing properties*, August 25, 1999

Proverbs 3:24-26

*"When you lie down, you will not be afraid;
when you lie down, your sleep will be sweet.
Have no fear of sudden disaster or
of the ruin that overtakes the wicked,
for the LORD will be your confidence
and will keep your foot from being snared."*

CHAPTER 22

MEDITATION

Jesus frequently sought a solitary place to spend time alone with God. According to Mark 1:35 [NIV]: *"Very early in the morning while it was still dark, Jesus got up, left the house, and went off to a solitary place where He prayed."*

Spending time with God, in silence and solitude, meditating on His Word, helps a person become physically healthier. It creates a sense of peace, joy, and contentment while allowing us to develop a stronger relationship with our Lord and Savior. Meditation has even been medically proven to reduce stress, and promote calm and a sense of inner peace...even eliminating or reducing the symptoms of many health issues.

Christian meditation is a form of prayer in which a

structured attempt is made to get in touch with and deliberately reflect on the revelations of God.[1] The word meditation comes from the Latin word *meditari* which means *to concentrate, to muse,* or *rehearse in one's mind.* Christian meditation is also the process of deliberately focusing on specific thoughts. Joshua 1:8 tells us to meditate on the Word of God day and night: ***"This book of the law shall not depart out of thy mouth; but thou shalt meditate therin day and night, that thou mayest observe to do according to all that is written therein: for then thou shalt make thy way prosperous, and then thou shalt have good success."***

Meditation refocuses us from ourselves and the world around us to reflect on God's Word, His nature, His abilities, and His works. Christians are to reflect on God's Word, which is ***"God-breathed and is useful for teaching, rebuking, correcting and training in righteousness, so that the man of God may be thoroughly equipped for every good work"*** [2 Timothy 3:16-17].

Christian meditation has nothing to do with practices that have Eastern mysticism as their foundation.

---

1. *Christian Meditation for Beginners* by Thomas Zanzig, Marilyn Kielbasa, 2000 ISBN 0884893618, page 7

Unlike eastern meditation practices whose purpose is to empty oneself of daily concerns, the Christian is seeking a closer experience, or relationship, with God as portrayed in the verse: ***"Be still and know that I am God"*** Psalm 46:10, (KJV)

The only true path to peace and fulfillment is through God. Isaiah 26:3 tells us: ***"You will keep in perfect peace him whose mind is steadfast, because he trusts in you."*** James 4:8 tells us: ***"Draw near to God and He will draw near to you."***

Take time to be alone, quiet, and listen—God can then speak into our minds. When God puts an idea into our mind, we call it *inspiration.* During meditation, we ask God to give us understanding through the Holy Spirit, Who has promised to lead us ***"Into all truth"*** John 16:13 Romans 12:2: tells us ***"And be not conformed to this world: but be ye transformed by the renewing of your mind, that ye may prove what is that good, and acceptable, and perfect, will of God."*** Ephesians 4:23: ***"be renewed in the spirit of your mind."***

When these basic requirements for health are provided and we keep our focus on God's will for our life, the self-healing mechanisms of our body attempt to restore and/or optimize our health. Our body's ability to heal itself and restore energy and vitality are a gift from God. The Apostle John states in 3 John 1:2: *"Beloved, I wish above all things that thou mayest prosper and be in health, even as thy soul prospereth."*

Leviticus 17:14

For it is the life of all flesh.
Its blood sustains its life.

CHAPTER 23

OUR BODY'S pH LEVEL AND HOW IT EFFECTS OUR HEALTH

pH is the abbreviation for **potential Hydrogen**. The higher the pH reading, the more alkaline and oxygen- rich our blood is. The lower the pH reading, the more acidic and oxygen-deprived our blood is. If a person has cancer, their pH reading will be very acidic or a bright yellow on the test paper.

0 1 2 3 4 5 6 7 **healthy** 8 9 10 11 12 13 14

Our blood stays in a very narrow pH range (right around 7.35 - 7.45). Below or above this range means symptoms and disease.[1] The Bible emphasizes just how important our blood is in Leviticus 17:11 *For the life of the flesh is in the blood...*

1. Lark, Susan, Dr., *Health and pH*

Saliva pH: You can test your pH simply by wetting a piece of litmus paper with your saliva. You can purchase pH strips or litmus paper online or at most health food stores. The best time to check your saliva pH is two hours after a meal, or upon arising before anything has been put into your mouth. A reading lower than 6.4 is indicative of insufficient alkaline reserves. If this occurs, the body has alkaline mineral deficiencies (mainly, calcium and magnesium) and will not assimilate food very well. **To deviate from ideal salivary pH for an extended time invites illness.**[2]

Acidosis is when your body remains in an acid pH state for an extended period of time. This can result in:

Rheumatoid arthritis	Lupus tuberculosis
high blood pressure	most cancers
anxiety	diarrhea dilated pupils
fatigue in early morning	headaches
hyperactivity	hyper-sexuality
nervousness	rapid heart beat
restless leg syndrome s	shortness of breath
strong cravings for sweets	dry hands and feet
diabetes	osteoporosis
insomnia	

2. http://www.falconblanco.com/health/alimentation/ph.htm

In order to balance your pH, the diet should focus on fresh raw fruits, vegetables, and mineral water and eliminate strong acidifiers such as sodas, wheat, white sugar, and limit red meat consumption. One of the best ways to raise one's body pH is by making sure that adequate minerals, particularly calcium, are present. In general, green vegetables are high in calcium. Kale, broccoli, and collard greens are good sources of calcium.

Urinary pH Test: The pH of the urine indicates how the body is working to maintain the proper pH of the blood. **Do not** test your urinary pH first thing in the morning, because your body is less hydrated after a night's rest, causing the reading to be more acidic. It is best to test your urinary pH at least two hours **after** a meal. The pH of urine indicates the efforts of the body via the kidneys, adrenals, lungs, and gonads to regulate pH through the buffer salts and hormones. The ideal pH range is 5.8 to 6.8.[3]

If your urinary pH stays too low, the diet should focus on foods considered to be alkaline-forming and thus helpful to people with consistently acid pH.

---

3. http://www.alkalizeforhealth.net/salivaphtest.htm

These include:

Almonds *(raw)*	aloe vera	apple
apricots	beans	bee pollen
buckwheat	cabbage	cantaloupe
celery	carrots	cucumbers
dairy products *(except hard cheese)*		goat's milk
dates	dulse	eggs *(poached)*
figs	grapefruit	honey
lemons	lettuce	millet
mineral water	miso soup	parsley
raisins	brown rice	peaches
red potatoes	pineapple	sprouted seeds
spinach *(cooked)*	turnip tops	

CHAPTER 24

ALKALINE-FORMING FOODS

Balanced pH is critical for human health. Consuming an excessive amount of highly acidic foods and beverages, emotional stress, and toxic overload caused by an impaired immune system will cause our body's pH to become acidic: an imbalance in the pH of your body is the precursor to illness and disease.

One method the body uses to restore proper pH balance is to pull alkaline minerals out of our bones—which are great storehouses of calcium and other alkaline minerals—and use those minerals to neutralize the acidic foods and beverages that have been consumed. The consumption of soft drinks is well-known to cause the depletion of minerals from the body's bones. This results in loss of bone mass density and the onset of osteoporosis. The more soft drinks a person consumes—the weaker their bones become.

High-protein/low-carbohydrate diets are also highly acidic, because red meats are very acidic. That is why a percentage of the weight loss on a nutritionally poor, low-carbohydrate diet actually results from loss of bone mass *not* loss of body fat!

Another way the body attempts to neutralize excess dietary acids is by increasing respirations, because carbon dioxide is acidic and oxygen is alkaline. By breathing in more oxygen and exhaling more carbon dioxide, the body works to regulate its own pH.[4]

When our pH level remains acidic for an extended period of time, it will: Decrease the body's ability to absorb minerals and other nutrients decrease the cell's energy production, decrease the cell's ability to repair damage, decrease the body's ability to detoxify heavy metals, which make tumor cells thrive makes a person more susceptible to fatigue and illness.

The main cause of acidosis is one's diet. If it is too high in acid-producing animal products like meat, eggs and dairy products, and processed foods like white flour, refined white sugar, and acid-producing beverages like coffee and soft drinks, your system will become unbalanced.

4. http://www.chlorellafactor.com/chlorella-spirulina

In order to restore one's body to a healthy balance, more alkaline-producing foods like fresh fruits and vegetables, and whole grains and legumes need to be added to one's daily diet.[5]

Another culprit that causes excess acidity is the consumption of large quantities of acid-producing prescription and over-the-counter drugs. These are very acid forming. A third cause of acidity is the excess use of artificial chemical sweeteners like **NutraSweet, Spoonful, Sweet 'N Low, Equal,** or **Aspartame**—all of which are extremely acid-forming. Evidence suggests that *aspartame* is also linked to health problems, including headaches, gas, confusion, and brain tumors [Roberts, 1990; Olney and others, 1996].

If you have a health problem, most likely you are acidic. Research shows that unless the body's pH level is slightly alkaline, the body cannot heal itself. So, no matter what type of treatment you choose to use to take care of your health problem, it won't be effective until your pH level is balanced. If your body's pH is not balanced, you cannot effectively assimilate vitamins, minerals, and food supplements. Your body's pH affects everything.

---

5. Sinclair, Jack, *Alkalize or Die – Here's Why!* May 19, 2010

Research has proven that disease [even cancer] *cannot survive* in an alkaline environment; however, disease and cancer cells *thrive* in an acidic, oxygen-deprived environment.

There are two factors that are *ALWAYS* present with cancer, no matter what else may be present. These two factors are: **Acid pH** and **lack of oxygen**. Cancer cells cannot survive in an oxygen-rich environment. Cancer and *all* diseases hate oxygen / pH balance. The proper alkalinity pH of the blood (7.35 - 7.45) is critical for the overall health of the body. Deuteronomy 12:23: *"... For the blood is the life..."*

One should also limit caffeinated and alcoholic drinks. These are diuretics and will dehydrate you.

Balancing the pH is a major step toward well-being and greater health. Acidosis (overly acidic body) is the primary indicator of Calcium Deficiency Disease. Scientists have discovered that the bodily fluids of healthy people are alkaline (high pH) whereas the bodily fluids of sick people are acidic (low pH). An acidic body is a sickness magnet.

To maintain health, the diet should consist of 60% alkaline-forming foods and 40% acid-forming foods. To restore health, the diet should consist of 80% alkaline-forming foods and 20% acid-forming foods.

If you are drinking diet soda which contains aspartame or using sugar-free products: diet sodas, foods labeled "sugarless," "sugar free," "diet food," "low calorie," and the like—you need to read the label to see if they contain ASPARTAME. Check labels carefully. Aspartame is extremely acid-forming and should be avoided.

Chapter 25

Dental Focus

Permanent Teeth

Maxillary Teeth
- Central incisor
- Lateral incisor
- Canine
- First premolar
- Second premolar
- First molar
- Second molar
- Third molar

Mandibular Teeth
- Third molar
- Second molar
- First molar
- Second premolar
- First premolar
- Canine
- Lateral incisor
- Central incisor

Several years ago, during my study of oriental medicine, I became aware of acupuncture meridians *and* how our teeth and body are interconnected. Our teeth can have a *direct* influence on the organs of our body. Each tooth is related to an acupuncture meridian which, in turn, is related to various organs, tissues, and glands throughout our body. These meridians are referred to as the "*energy highway*." The connection is *so obvious* that your overall health and wellness can be assessed by reviewing your dental condition.

I have never been able to have children and always wondered why? I thought I would have a dozen—I just love kids! What I found out about teeth, and their relationship with other organ systems, encouraged my continued research. I discovered that tooth #8, the first incisor, has direct association to conceptual connections, hormonal capacity, impotence, sterility, and a list of other health conditions.[1]

Wow! What a revelation!

On Christmas day 1970, my younger brother, Tommy, received a mini-bike. He just loved it, and it looked like so much fun—I just had to try it out myself.

---

1. American Bio-Compatible Health Systems, Inc. 2009. http://naturaldentistry.us/holistic-dentistry/meridian-tooth-chart-from-encinitas-dentist/

He allowed me the opportunity to drive it. It was great fun; however, when I decided to stop, I flew right over the handlebars and into the gravel, face first, knocking out my front tooth. Little did I know—that event when I was fourteen years old probably sealed my fate and prevented me from ever having children!

I also learned that root canals are harmful to one's overall health. Unfortunately, I already *had* two root canals; and because of the expense involved in having them removed, I never made extracting them a priority. ***Bad decision!*** The two teeth were: tooth #3 – the first molar, directly associated with the mammary gland on the left side of the body, and tooth #4 – the second premolar, related to the motility and peristalsis in the small and large intestine. Another revelation!

My history of chronic constipation could very well have been caused by the root canal I had done in

1972 when I was only sixteen. Then, sometime between 1995 and 1998, I had the second root canal done. That very well may have been what started the chain of events that finally led to breast cancer.

The evidence seems overwhelming. In my life, I have experienced three different dental problems and three different health conditions. The fact that the acupuncture meridians are linked from each of my problem teeth to the organ system that afflicted my body, proves to me that they are, in fact, interconnected. No one can convince me that this is just a coincidence.

Now that I had been diagnosed with cancer, my only solution was to have my root canals, my cap, and the dental amalgam removed from my teeth and replaced with all natural materials. There is a specialized type of dentist, a *"biological"* or *"holistic"* dentist—the only type that should be contacted for proper removal of root canals and replacement of caps and fillings. A biological dentist will use precautionary methods to prevent toxins from being released into the body and will use only natural and safe material.

If it had not been for the willingness of our friends to loan us the money for my treatment, I would not have been able to afford to have this vitally important but expensive dental work performed.

According to *The Independent Cancer Research Foundation*, root canals are a haven for microbes. No blood can reach the inside of the root canal, which prevents one's immune system from killing any microbes inside the dead tooth.[2]

2. http://www.new-cancer-treatments.org/Articles/RootCanals.html

Dr. Thomas Rau, who ran the Paracelsus Cancer Clinic in Switzerland since 1958, checked the records of 150 breast cancer patients treated in his clinic. He found that 147 of them (98%) had one or more root canal teeth on the same meridian as the original breast cancer tumor.

There are approximately twenty-four million root canals done in the U.S. every year. In a 1925 study conducted by Dr. Weston Price and sixty other prominent researchers, these dental procedures were proven to be deadly disease agents. That study has been suppressed since that time by the ***American Dental Association*** [ADA] and the ***American Association of Endodontists*** (AAE).

George Meinig, DDS, FACD, an endodontist, helped found the AAE in 1943. After practicing his craft for fifty years, he retired in 1993. He discovered the Weston Price research shortly after his retirement and concluded there ***is no safe way*** to do a root canal filling. He wrote the book: ***Root Canal Cover-Up***—first published in 1994—as "*mea culpa*" to the thousands of patients whose health he ruined by doing root canals.

Author's Note:
I suggest you read Dr. Meinig's book for the full story.

He has also lectured widely since then trying to alert people to this extreme danger to their health. [3]

"I have had a number of patients with breast cancer, all of whom had root canals on the tooth related to the breast area on the associated energy meridian,' John Diamond, M.D.[4]

It is impossible to cure diseases unless all of the root canal teeth are removed properly by a Naturopathic or *biological* dentist because, even if you killed the microbes of the disease, the microbes hiding in the root canals can come out and re-infect the person! Cancer, some cases of Type One diabetes, and a host of other diseases are caused by microbes, viruses, bacteria, and fungi such as yeasts and molds. To cure these diseases, the microbes must be killed throughout the body so the immune system can restore the body to its normal state.[5]

---

3. http://v.mercola.com/blogs/public_blog/Cancer-Continues-to-"-Continues-to-Worsen-8023.aspx
4. John Diamond, M.D., Triad Medical Centre, 4600 Kietzke Lane, M-242, Reno, NV 89502. Tel: 775-829 2277
5. http://www.new-cancer-treatments.org/Articles/RootCanals.html

CHAPTER 26

COFFEE ENEMA CLEANSE

The enema has been called *"one of the oldest medical procedures still in use today."* The Egyptian *Ebers Papyrus* (*circa* 1550 B.C.), one of the oldest preserved medical documents known to be in existence, mentions it.

While serving as a medic in World War I, Max Gerson, M.D., found that utilizing coffee rather than water for enemas had hitherto unknown healing and pain-relieving benefits for wounded soldiers. The caffeine in coffee administered as an enema detoxifies the liver. It is a natural treatment for cancer and other degenerative diseases.

No matter which degenerative disease is causing symptoms, the coffee enema will offer relief from confusion, general nervous tension, depression, allergy-related symptoms, and most importantly, *severe pain.*[1]

1. Gerson and Walker, *"The Gerson Therapy"*

Once on the enema regimen, many people have noted a paradoxical calming effect, reduced stress, and an overall restorative feeling.

Organic coffee is a powerful agent for detoxifying. When used in enemas, it purifies the liver and its stored toxins.[2]

Since the enema is generally held for fifteen minutes, and all the blood in the body passes through the liver every three minutes, 'these enemas represent a form of dialysis of blood across the gut wall' (Healing Newsletter, #13, May-June, 1986). Leviticus 17:11 **...For the life of the body is in its blood...**

Dr. Lee Wattenberg was able to show that substances found in coffee—*kahweol* and *cafestol palmitate*—promote the activity of a key enzyme system, *glutathione S-transferase*. This system detoxifies a vast array of *electrophiles* [i.e. electron-lovers] from the bloodstream and is responsible for neutralizing *free radicals*—harmful chemicals now commonly implicated in the initiation of cancer. Joel 3:21: **"For I will cleanse their blood..."** According to Gar Hildenbrand of the *Gerson Institute*, coffee enemas *"must be regarded as an important mechanism for carcinogen detoxification."*

---

2. Mechelle, Marie, articledashboard.com, *Natural Cure For Breast Cancer With Coffee Enemas*

CHAPTER 27

BENEFITS OF A COFFEE ENEMA

- Aids in elimination of the liver's toxic wastes
- Stimulates the liver's production of enzymes that cleanse blood
- Draws out environmental and metabolic toxins
- Improves digestion and absorption of nutrients
- Cleanses the colon
- Improves the complexion
- Reduces puffiness around the eyes
- Improves joint health and flexibility
- Decreases congestion and allergies[1]

The coffee enema—combined with a diet rich in fresh organic juices, fruits and vegetables, and supplements—has proven an effective method for combating breast cancer.

1 Ball, Jeanne, coffee-enemas.blogspot.com, January 27, 2009

By flooding the body with nutrition while eliminating toxins, it boosts the body's cancer-fighting ability allowing it to heal naturally.

This treatment has so many health benefits that it should override any hesitation a person has to incorporate it into their regular hygiene program. The evidence is *overwhelming*—coffee enemas are an effective cure for cancer and many other serious health conditions. Traditional cancer treatment—chemotherapy, radiation, and drugs—are devastating to one's physical and mental health and their quality of life.

Although it is not easy to restore one's health after a serious condition has manifested itself—it *can* be done. There are countless reports and research proving that proper diet, exercise, mental attitude, detoxification, and faith in God's *healing power* is stronger than any disease.

Whether a person chooses to use this alternative approach to conventional medicine or simply as a supplement to help purify the system after chemotherapy, the coffee enema is a great cleanse that will help improve detoxification of your system.

CHAPTER 27

REFERENCES AND CITATIONS

Source obtained from the internet:
naturaldentistry.us/holistic-dentistry/meridian-tooth-chart-from-encinitas-dentist/
Source obtained from the internet:
naturaldentistry.us/tag/acupuncture-meridian/
Source obtained from the internet:
extoxnet.orst.edu/faqs/dietcancer/homepage/cancer-prevention.html
Source obtained from the internet:
beating-cancer-gently.com/ FreeNewsletter
Source obtained from the internet:
cdc.gov/sleep/chronic_disease.htm
Source obtained from the internet:
allaboutspirituality.org/Christian-meditation-fq.htm
Source obtained from the internet:
thechristianmediator.com/
Source obtained from the internet:
new-cancer-treatments.or/Articles/ RootCanals.html
Source obtained from the internet:
Articledashboard.com/Article/ Natural-Cure-for-

Breast-Cancer-with-Coffee-Enemas/686057
Annemarie Colbin, *Aspartame: The Real Story*, by X
Source obtained from the internet:
foodandhealing.com/articles/article- aspartame.htm
Source obtained from the internet:
indigo.com/test-strips/ph-test-strips. html
Source obtained from the internet:
alkalizeforhealth.net/salivaphtest. htm
Source obtained from the internet: **snopes.com/medical/ toxins/aspartame.asp**
Source obtained from the internet:
alkalizeforhealth.net/rebounder.htm
Source obtained from the internet:
psychologydebunked.com/ email0802_prescriptiondrugdeaths.htm
Source obtained from the internet:
scribd.com/doc/6635922/Natural- Cancer-Treatments
Source obtained from the internet:
townsendletter.com/Dec2007/
Source obtained from the internet:
forbes.com/2009/07/07/healthiest-foods-nutrition-lifestyle-health-heathiest-foods.html
Source obtained from the internet:
cmaj.ca/cgi/content/full/171/12/1451
Source obtained from the internet:
campaignfortruth.com/ Eclub/200202/overdose.htm
Source obtained from the internet:
4.dr-rath-foundation.org/THE_ FOUNDATION/ News/2010/pharmaceutical_business/index.htm
Source obtained from the internet:
alternativehealth.co.nz/cancer/index.htm

Reports from the University of Toronto (Clin Chim Acta, 235: 2, 1995 Mar 31, 207-19)
Respected cancer researcher, Ralph Moss, wrote enthusiastically about *The Grape Cure* in the Spring, 1997, issue of his Media Watch
Source obtained from the internet:
mayoclinic.com/health/red-wine/ HB00089
Source obtained from the internet:
winetastingguy.com/
Source obtained from the internet:
marksdailyapple.com/the-worlds-healthiest-countries
Source: U.S. National Institutes of Health, National Cancer Institute
Source obtained from the internet:
medicinenet.com/cancer/page2.htm
Source obtained from the internet:
busywomensfitness.com/exercise- benefits.html
Source obtained from the internet:
ctds.info/5_13_magnesium.html
Dietary Reference Intakes for Water, Potassium, Sodium, Chloride, and Sulfate, available at **nap.edu**
National Academies News Release:
Report Sets Dietary Levels for Water, Salt, and Potassium to Maintain Health and Reduce Chronic Disease Risk, February 11, 2004, available at 8.nationalacademies.org/ onpinews/ newsitem.aspx?RecordID=10925
Jane E. Brody, *Must I Have Another Glass? Maybe Not*, a New Report Says, N.Y. Times, February 17, 2004
Water and Nutrient-Rich Foods, The Sensible Way to Top Up Your Daily Water Requirement, available at **brita.net/water_and_nutrient_ rich_foods.html**

Dian A Dooley, Ph.D., *Water, Water Everywhere*, available at i**slandscene.com/Article.aspx?id=2472**
Molly Siple, *Juicy Foods: Need Fluid Fast? Drink Water. Otherwise, Foods With a High Water Content Can Provide Taste, Texture and Variety as They Contribute to Your Body's Reservoir*,
Source obtained from the internet: **findarticles.com/p/articles/mi_m0876/is_n51/ai_8540811/**
Diuretics cause magnesium loss
Source obtained from the internet: **holisticmed.com/aspartame/recent. html**
Source obtained from the internet: **wired.com/science/discoveries/ news/2002/10/56072, Pancreatic Cancer treated with twice daily coffee enemas**
Source obtained from the internet: **thoughtscreate.com/abccompete. html (E-book)**
Source obtained from the internet: life. **gaiamcom/gaiam/p/10WaystoDetoxifyYourBody.html**
Source obtained from the internet: **healingcancernaturally.com/thoughts-create-reality-links.html**
Source obtained from the internet: **healingcancernaturally.com/heal- yourself-with-mind-power.html**
Source obtained from the internet: **cancer.suite101.com/article.cfm/does-chrysanthemum-extract-cure-cancer**
Source obtained from the internet: **healingdeva.com/coffee_enemas. htm**
Source obtained from the internet: **cancerfightingstrategies.com**

Murray, M. and Pizzorno, J. *Encyclopedia of Natural Medicine.* (1998). Rocklin, CA Prima Publishing.

Carper, J. (1988). *The Food Pharmacy.* New York: Bantam Books

Hausman, P. & Benn Hurley, J. (1989). *The Healing Foods.* Emmaus, Pennsylvania: Rodale Press

Duke, J.A. (1997). *The Green Pharmacy.* Emmaus, Pennsylvania: Rodale Press

For more information on ordering books

or

if you would like to contact

Karen Drake, D. Min., T.M.D.

to speak at your event please contact:

karen@phxut.us

Phoenix University of Theology International

PO Box 86054

Phoenix, AZ 85080

USA

Made in the USA
Charleston, SC
08 September 2015